I0706965

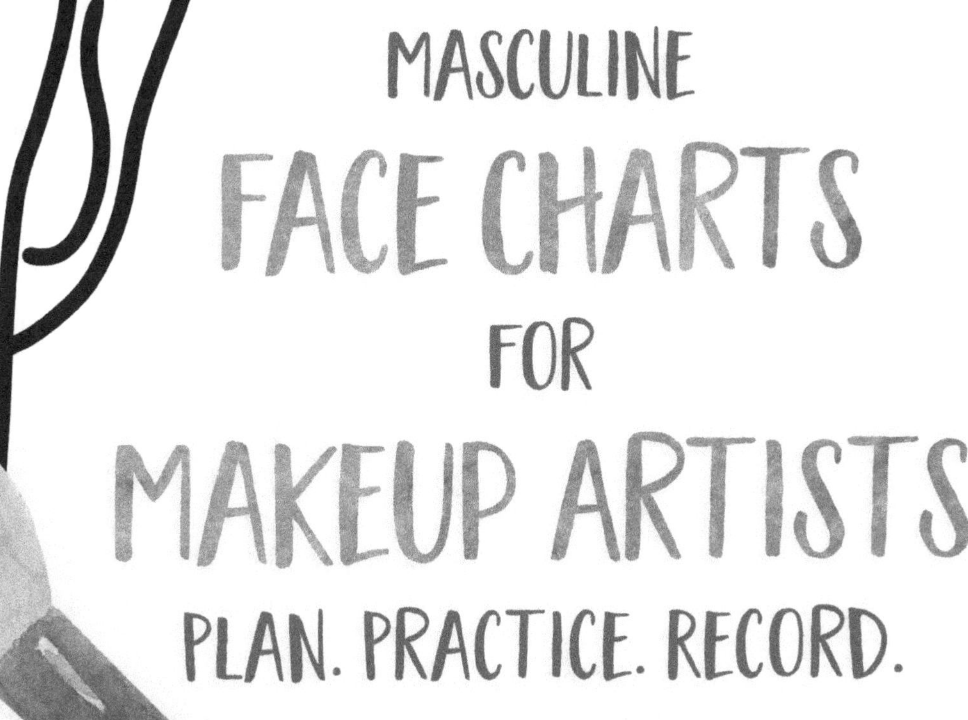

MASCULINE
FACE CHARTS
FOR
MAKEUP ARTISTS
PLAN. PRACTICE. RECORD.

ISBN: 978-1651395059

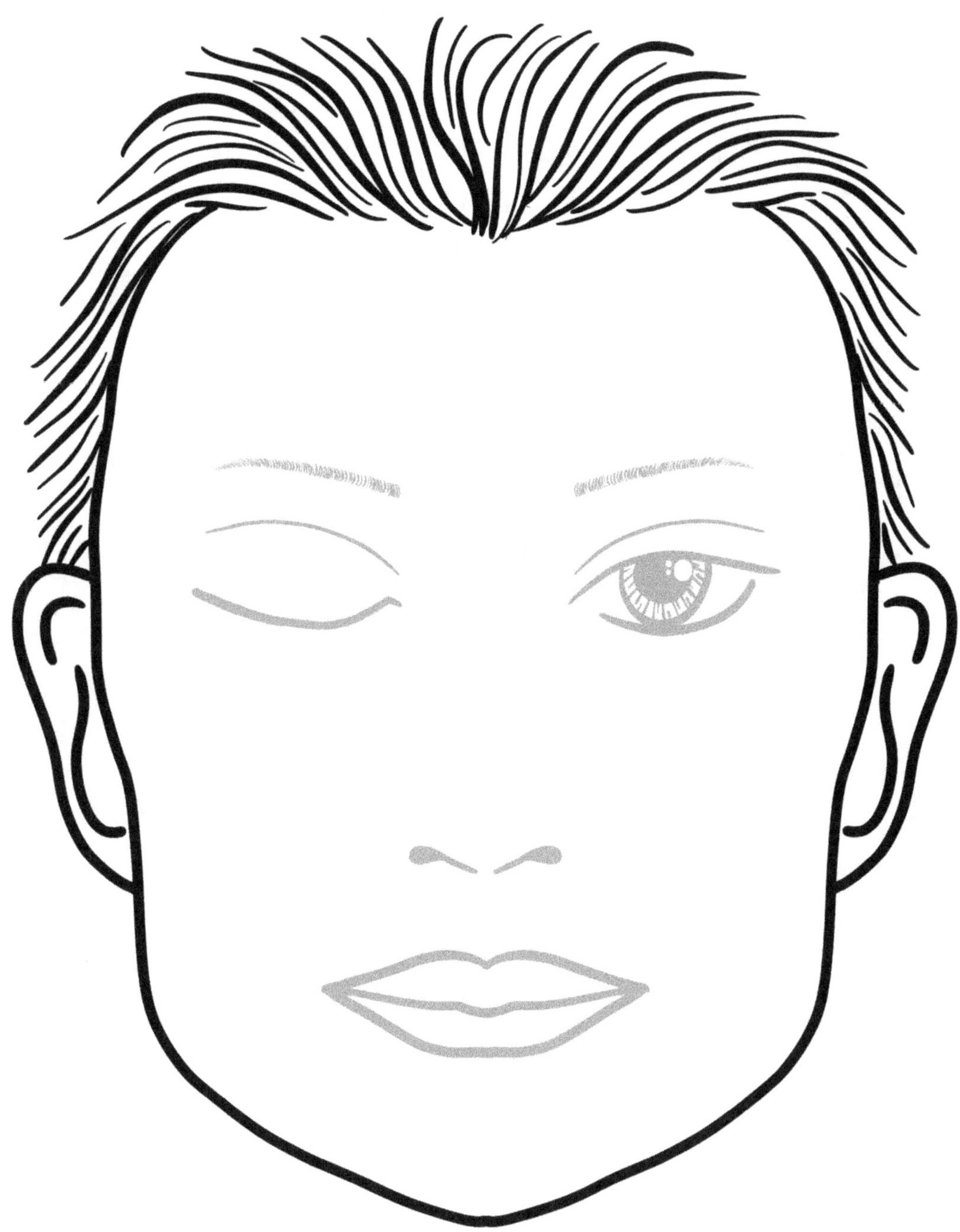

Details

Skin Tone _______________________

Eye Color _______________________

Hair Color _______________________

Lips (color, brand, etc.)

Lip Liner _______________________

Lip Color _______________________

Gloss _______________________

Eyes (color, brand, etc.)

Brows _______________________

Lid Color 1 _______________________

Lid Color 2 _______________________

Lid Color 3 _______________________

Crease _______________________

Eye Liner _______________________

Mascara _______________________

Face (color, brand, etc.)

Concealer _______________________

Foundation _______________________

Contour _______________________

Blush _______________________

Highlights _______________________

Powder _______________________

Date _______________________

Design/Client Name _______________________

	Concealer	Foundation	Contour	Blush	Highlights	Powder	Eye Liner	Mascara
	Brows	Lid Color 1	Lid Color 2	Lid Color 3	Crease	Lip Liner	Lip Color	Lip Gloss

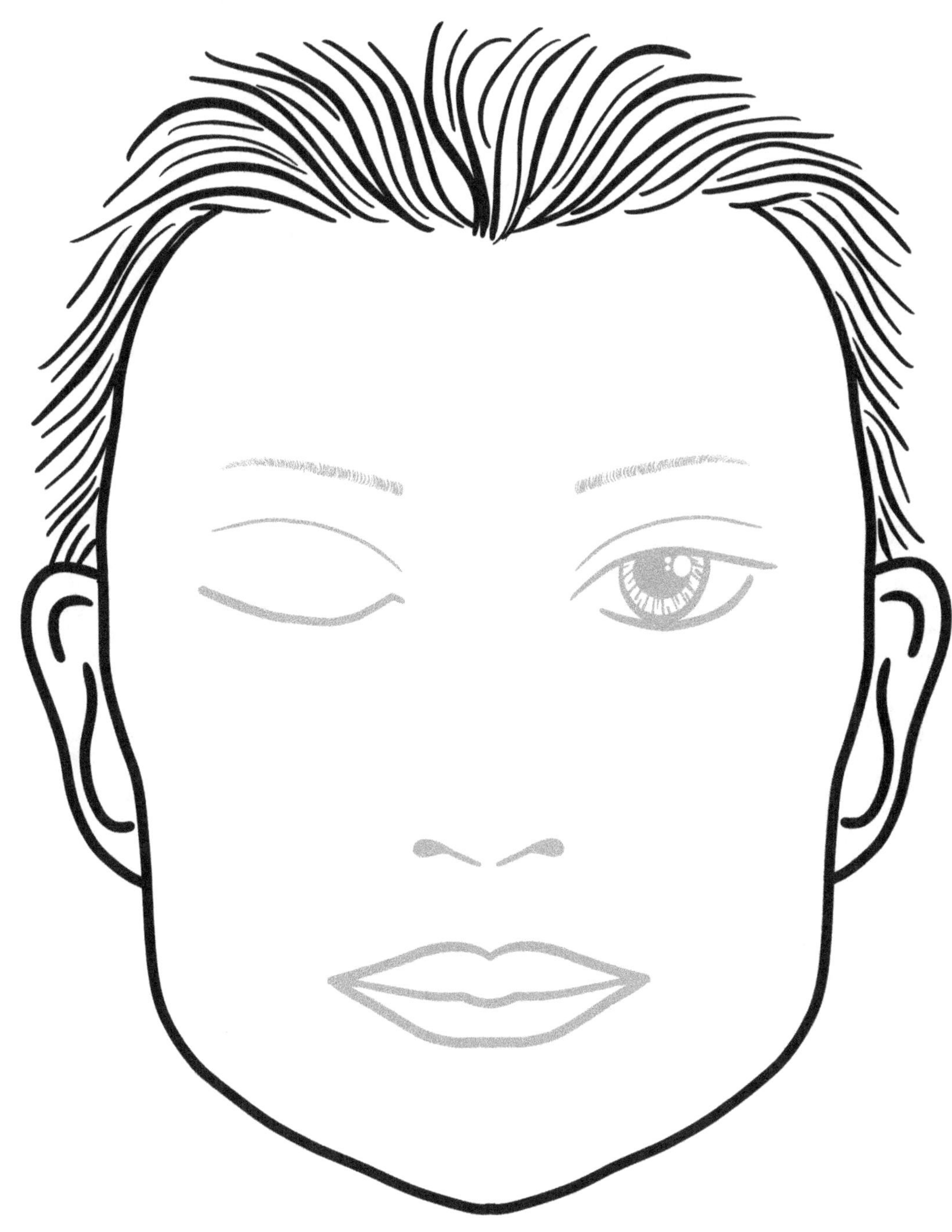

Details

Skin Tone______________________

Eye Color ______________________

Hair Color______________________

Lips (color, brand, etc.)

Lip Liner ______________________

Lip Color ______________________

Gloss ______________________

Eyes (color, brand, etc.)

Brows ______________________

Lid Color 1 ______________________

Lid Color 2 ______________________

Lid Color 3 ______________________

Crease______________________

Eye Liner______________________

Mascara ______________________

Face (color, brand, etc.)

Concealer______________________

Foundation______________________

Contour______________________

Blush ______________________

Highlights ______________________

Powder______________________

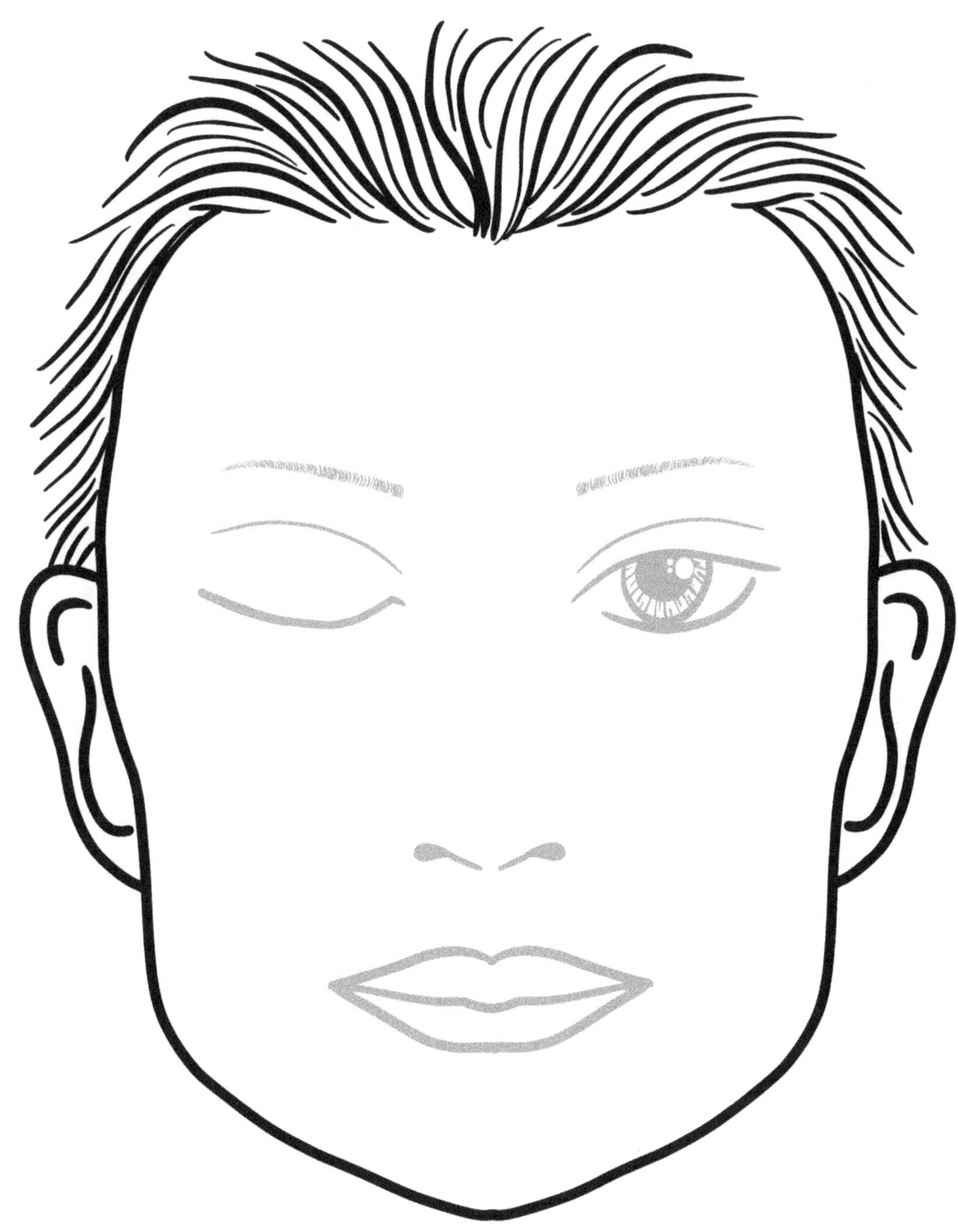

Details

Skin Tone _______________________

Eye Color _______________________

Hair Color _______________________

Lips (color, brand, etc.)

Lip Liner _______________________

Lip Color _______________________

Gloss _______________________

Eyes (color, brand, etc.)

Brows _______________________

Lid Color 1 _______________________

Lid Color 2 _______________________

Lid Color 3 _______________________

Crease _______________________

Eye Liner _______________________

Mascara _______________________

Face (color, brand, etc.)

Concealer _______________________

Foundation _______________________

Contour _______________________

Blush _______________________

Highlights _______________________

Powder _______________________

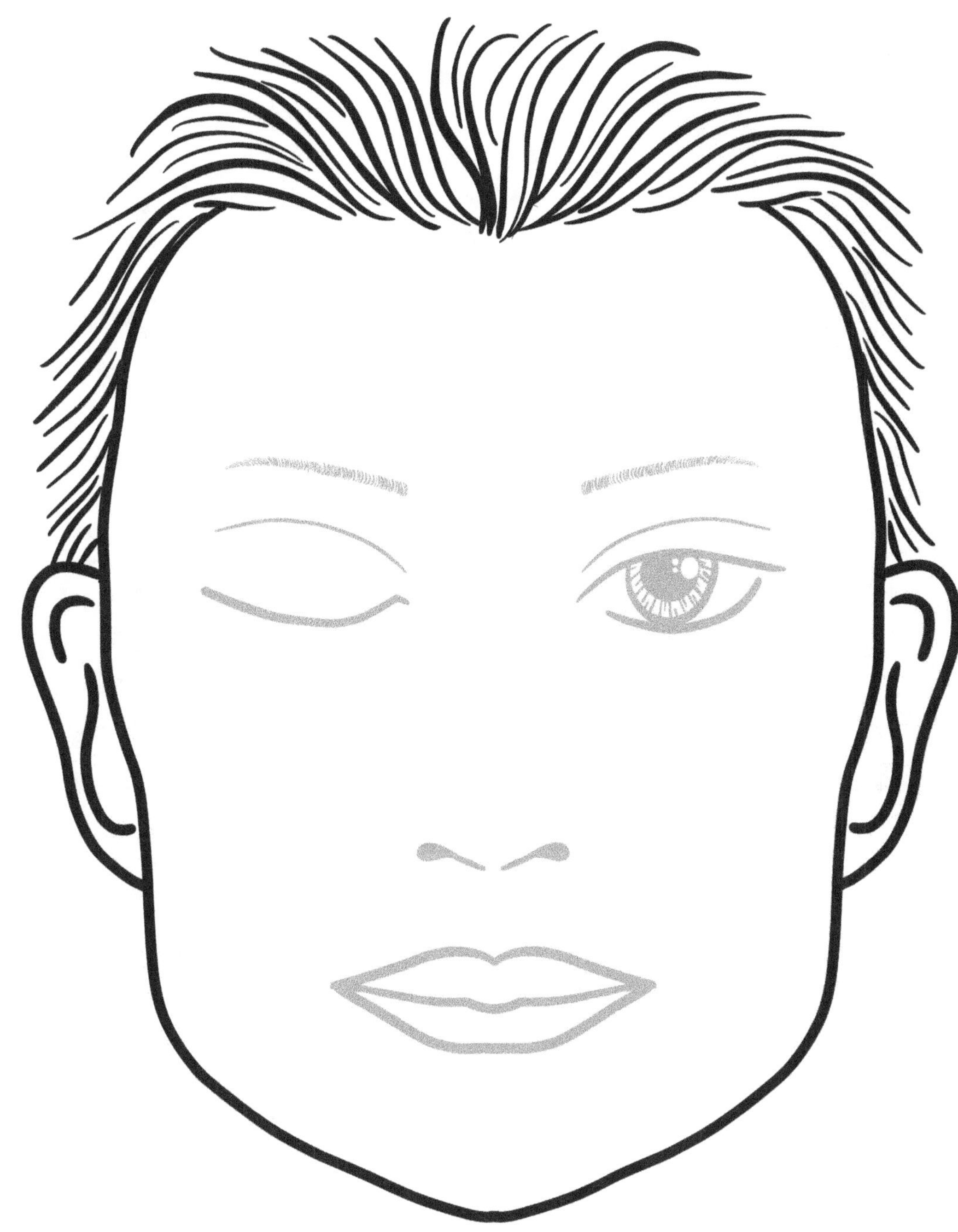

Details

Skin Tone __________________

Eye Color __________________

Hair Color __________________

Lips (color, brand, etc.)

Lip Liner __________________

Lip Color __________________

Gloss __________________

Eyes (color, brand, etc.)

Brows __________________

Lid Color 1 __________________

Lid Color 2 __________________

Lid Color 3 __________________

Crease __________________

Eye Liner __________________

Mascara __________________

Face (color, brand, etc.)

Concealer __________________

Foundation __________________

Contour __________________

Blush __________________

Highlights __________________

Powder __________________

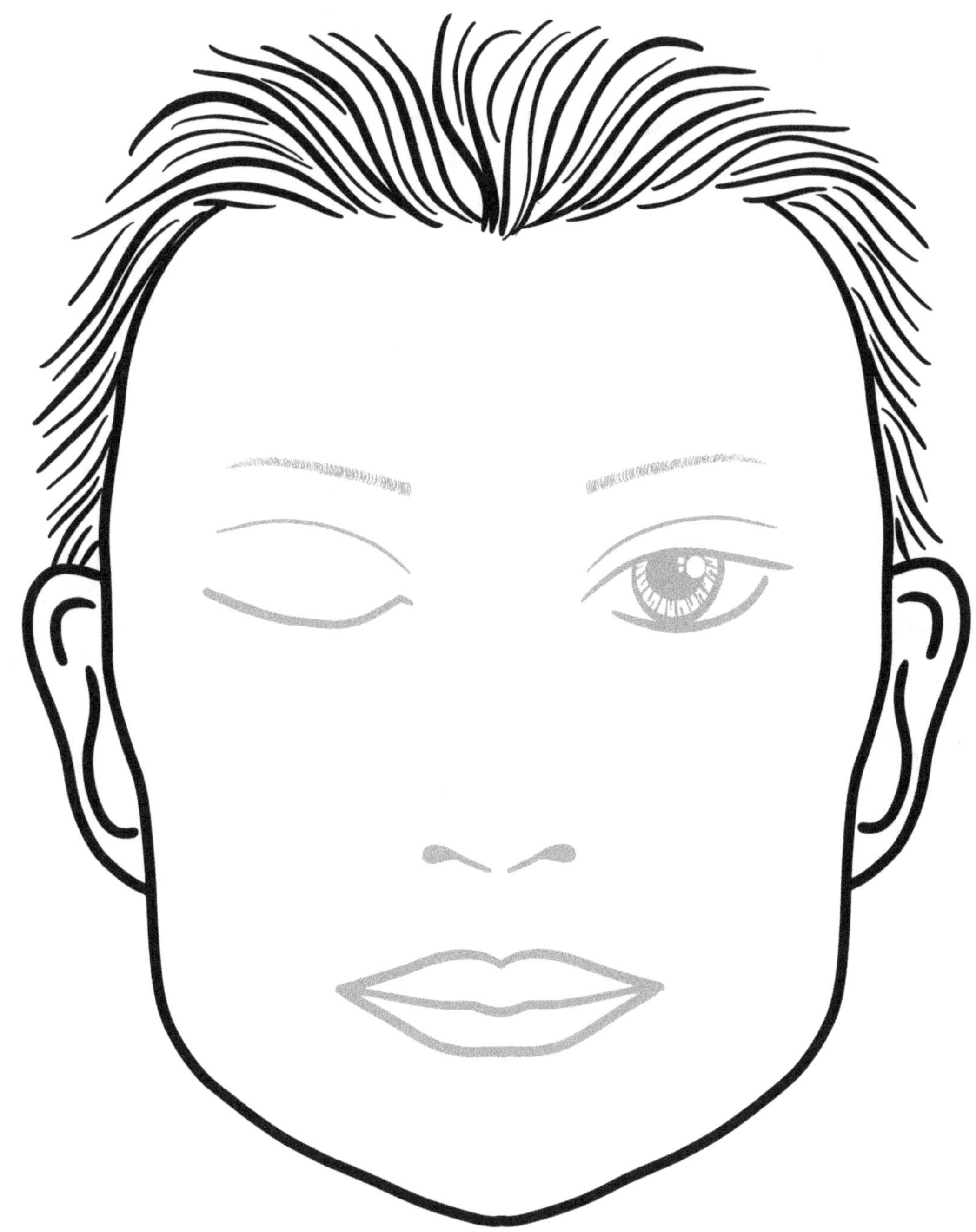

Details

Skin Tone _____________________

Eye Color _____________________

Hair Color _____________________

Lips (color, brand, etc.)

Lip Liner _____________________

Lip Color _____________________

Gloss _____________________

Eyes (color, brand, etc.)

Brows _____________________

Lid Color 1 _____________________

Lid Color 2 _____________________

Lid Color 3 _____________________

Crease _____________________

Eye Liner _____________________

Mascara _____________________

Face (color, brand, etc.)

Concealer _____________________

Foundation _____________________

Contour _____________________

Blush _____________________

Highlights _____________________

Powder _____________________

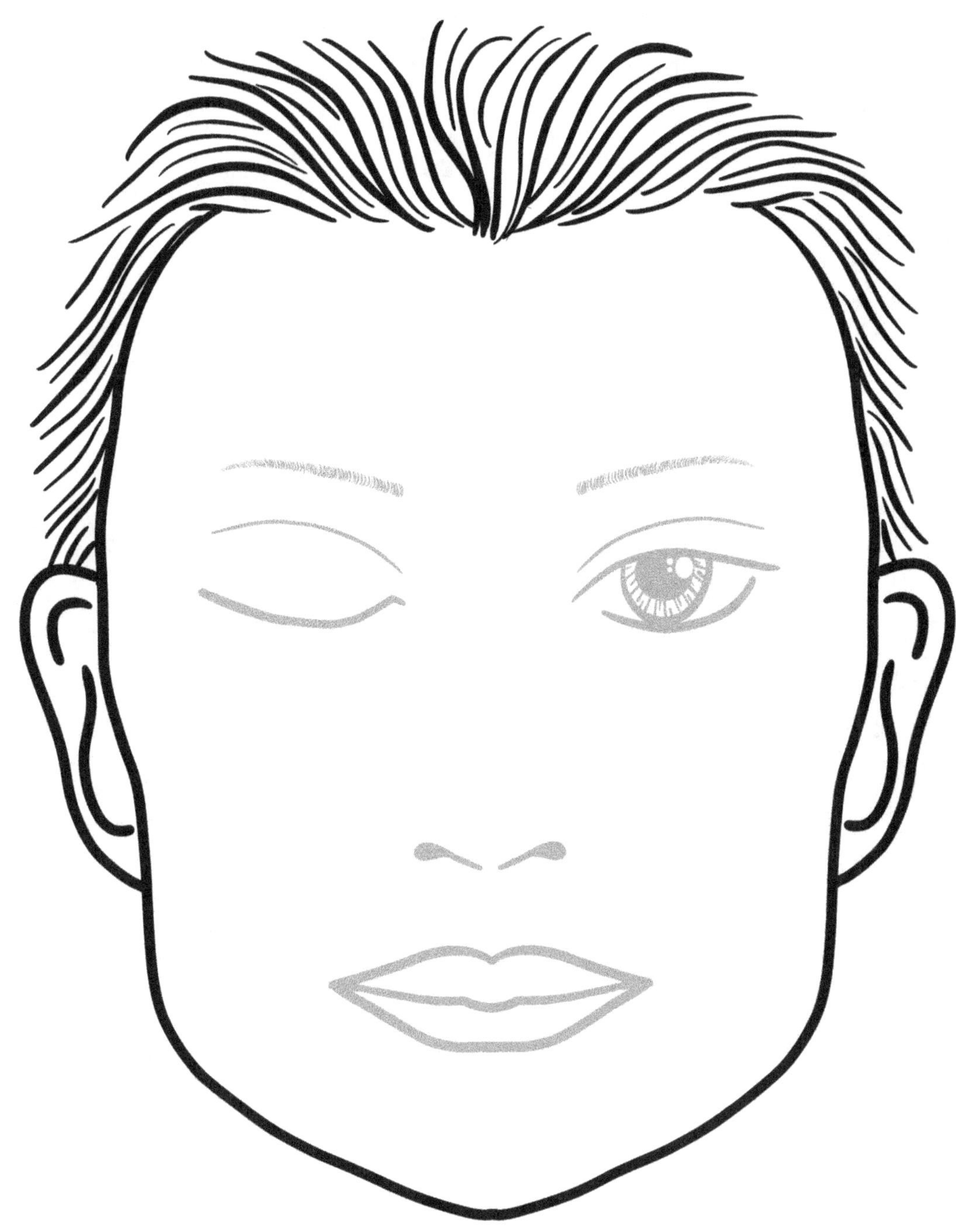

Details

Skin Tone _______________

Eye Color _______________

Hair Color _______________

Lips (color, brand, etc.)

Lip Liner _______________

Lip Color _______________

Gloss _______________

Eyes (color, brand, etc.)

Brows _______________

Lid Color 1 _______________

Lid Color 2 _______________

Lid Color 3 _______________

Crease _______________

Eye Liner _______________

Mascara _______________

Face (color, brand, etc.)

Concealer _______________

Foundation _______________

Contour _______________

Blush _______________

Highlights _______________

Powder _______________

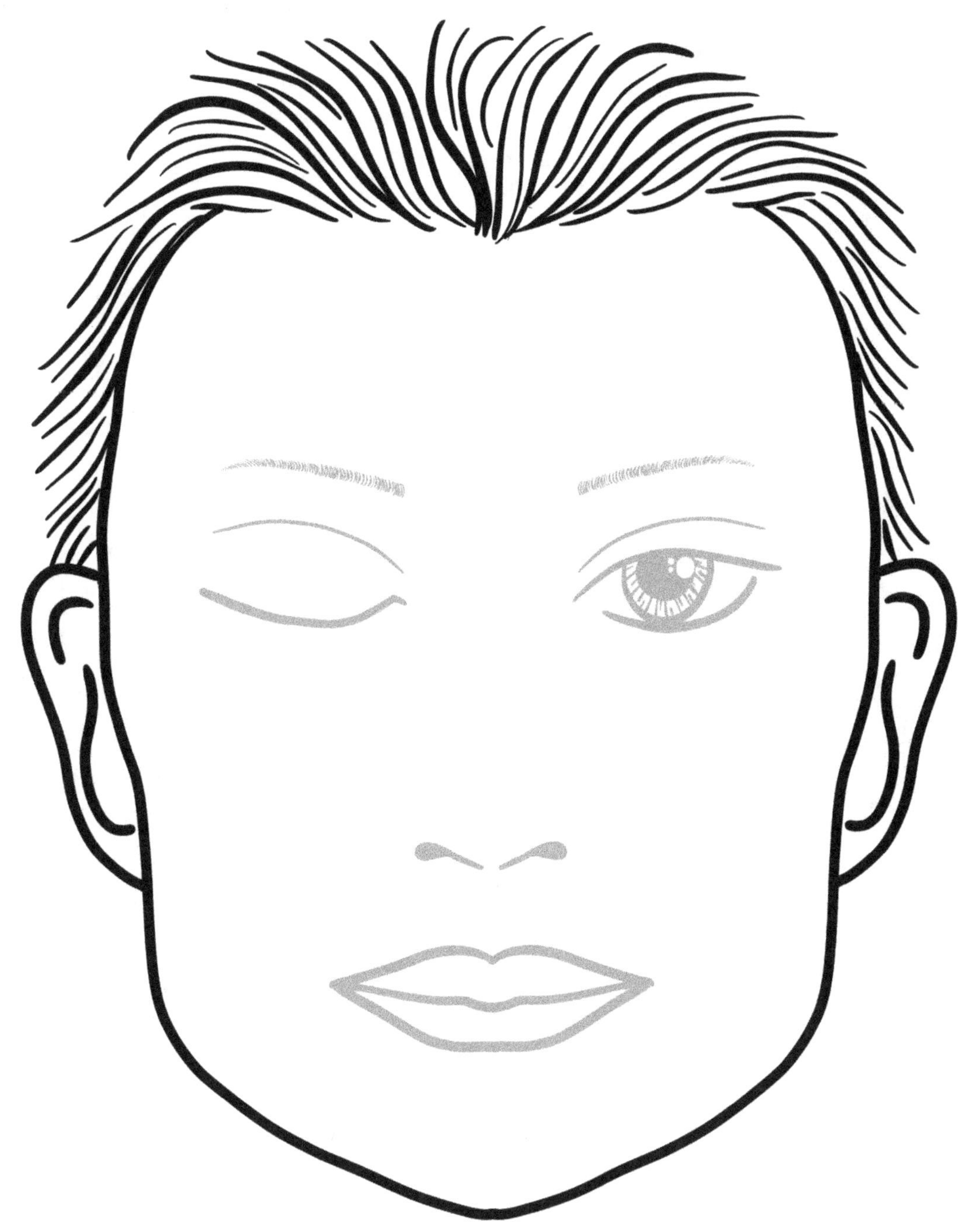

Date ___________

Design/Client Name ___________

Mascara	Lip Gloss
Eye Liner	Lip Color
Powder	Lip Liner
Highlights	Crease
Blush	Lid Color 3
Contour	Lid Color 2
Foundation	Lid Color 1
Concealer	Brows

Details

Skin Tone ___________________

Eye Color ___________________

Hair Color ___________________

Lips (color, brand, etc.)

Lip Liner ___________________

Lip Color ___________________

Gloss ___________________

Eyes (color, brand, etc.)

Brows ___________________

Lid Color 1 ___________________

Lid Color 2 ___________________

Lid Color 3 ___________________

Crease ___________________

Eye Liner ___________________

Mascara ___________________

Face (color, brand, etc.)

Concealer ___________________

Foundation ___________________

Contour ___________________

Blush ___________________

Highlights ___________________

Powder ___________________

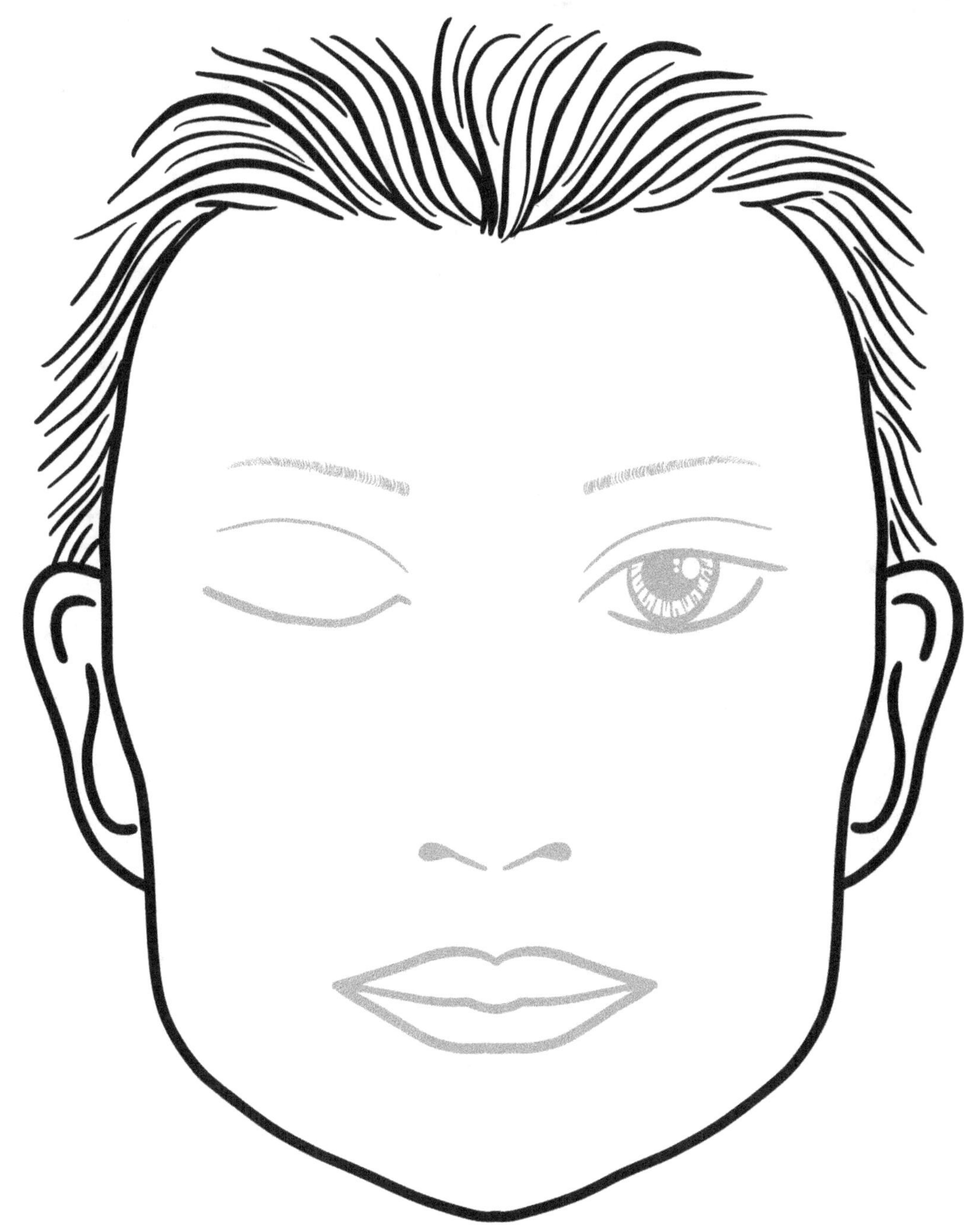

Details

Skin Tone ___________________

Eye Color ___________________

Hair Color ___________________

Lips (color, brand, etc.)

Lip Liner ___________________

Lip Color ___________________

Gloss ___________________

Eyes (color, brand, etc.)

Brows ___________________

Lid Color 1 ___________________

Lid Color 2 ___________________

Lid Color 3 ___________________

Crease ___________________

Eye Liner ___________________

Mascara ___________________

Face (color, brand, etc.)

Concealer ___________________

Foundation ___________________

Contour ___________________

Blush ___________________

Highlights ___________________

Powder ___________________

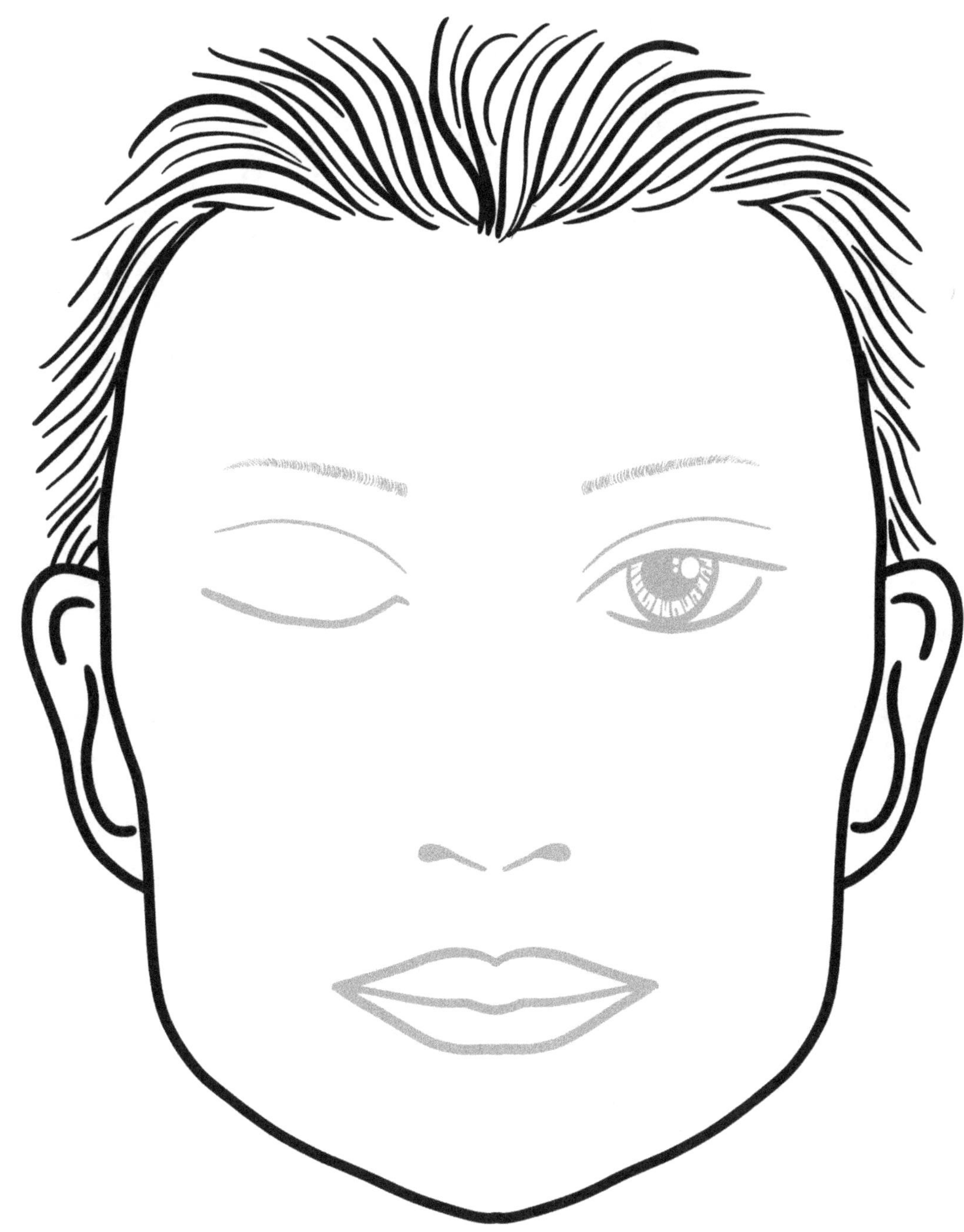

Details

Skin Tone _____________________

Eye Color _____________________

Hair Color _____________________

Lips (color, brand, etc.)

Lip Liner _____________________

Lip Color _____________________

Gloss _____________________

Eyes (color, brand, etc.)

Brows _____________________

Lid Color 1 _____________________

Lid Color 2 _____________________

Lid Color 3 _____________________

Crease _____________________

Eye Liner _____________________

Mascara _____________________

Face (color, brand, etc.)

Concealer _____________________

Foundation _____________________

Contour _____________________

Blush _____________________

Highlights _____________________

Powder _____________________

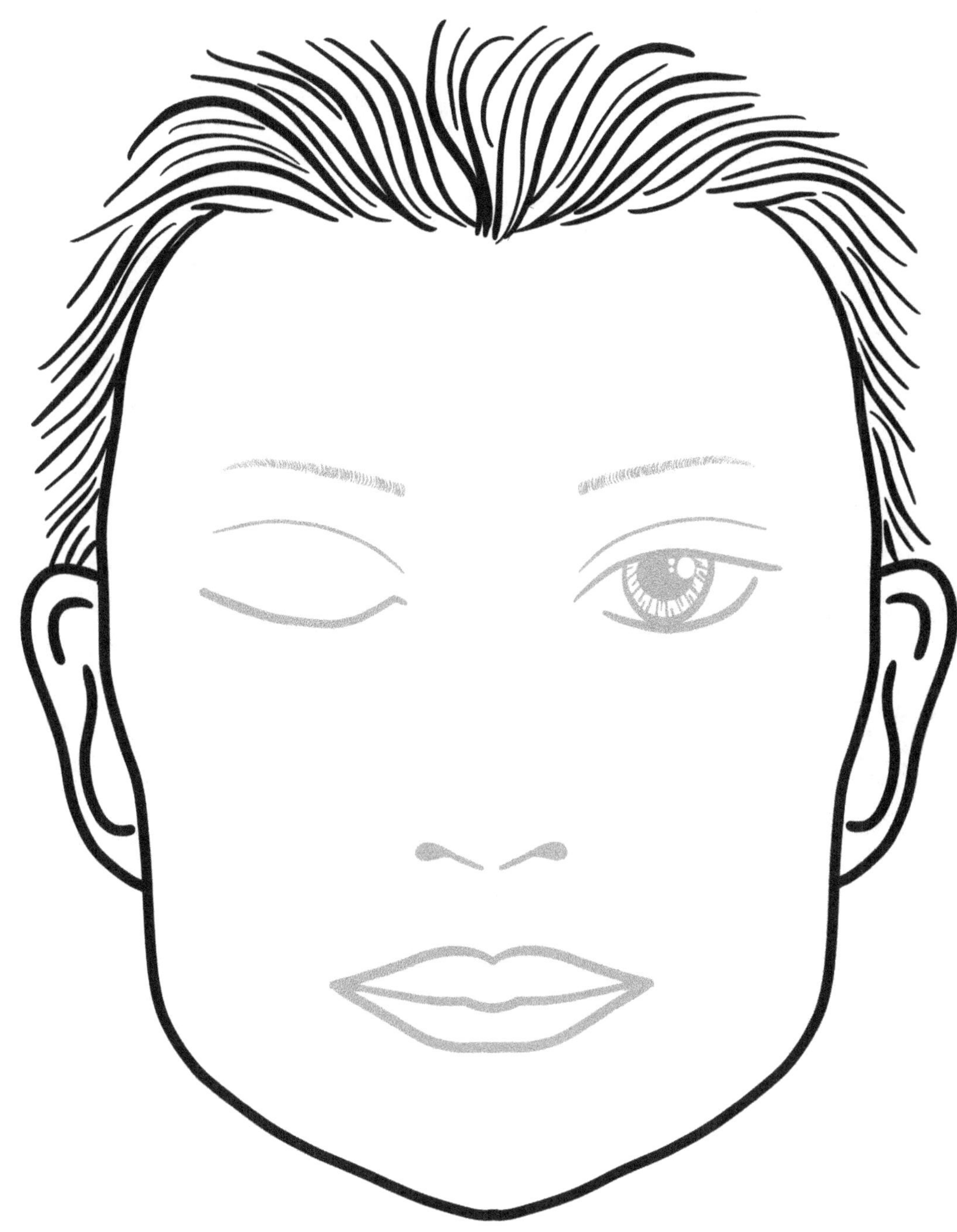

Details

Skin Tone _____________________

Eye Color _____________________

Hair Color _____________________

Lips (color, brand, etc.)

Lip Liner _____________________

Lip Color _____________________

Gloss _____________________

Eyes (color, brand, etc.)

Brows _____________________

Lid Color 1 _____________________

Lid Color 2 _____________________

Lid Color 3 _____________________

Crease _____________________

Eye Liner _____________________

Mascara _____________________

Face (color, brand, etc.)

Concealer _____________________

Foundation _____________________

Contour _____________________

Blush _____________________

Highlights _____________________

Powder _____________________

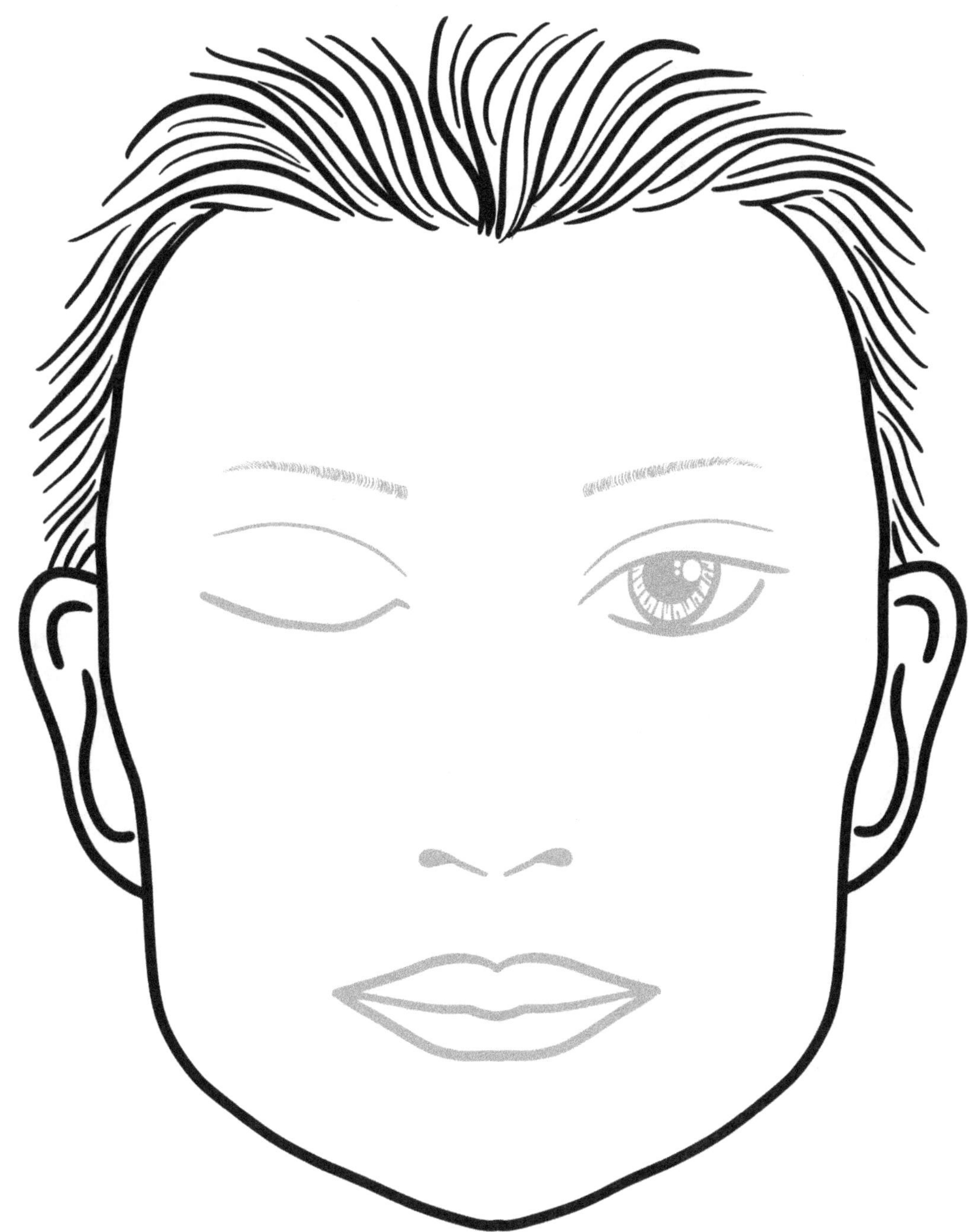

Details

Skin Tone _______________________

Eye Color _______________________

Hair Color _______________________

Lips (color, brand, etc.)

Lip Liner _______________________

Lip Color _______________________

Gloss _______________________

Eyes (color, brand, etc.)

Brows _______________________

Lid Color 1 _______________________

Lid Color 2 _______________________

Lid Color 3 _______________________

Crease _______________________

Eye Liner _______________________

Mascara _______________________

Face (color, brand, etc.)

Concealer _______________________

Foundation _______________________

Contour _______________________

Blush _______________________

Highlights _______________________

Powder _______________________

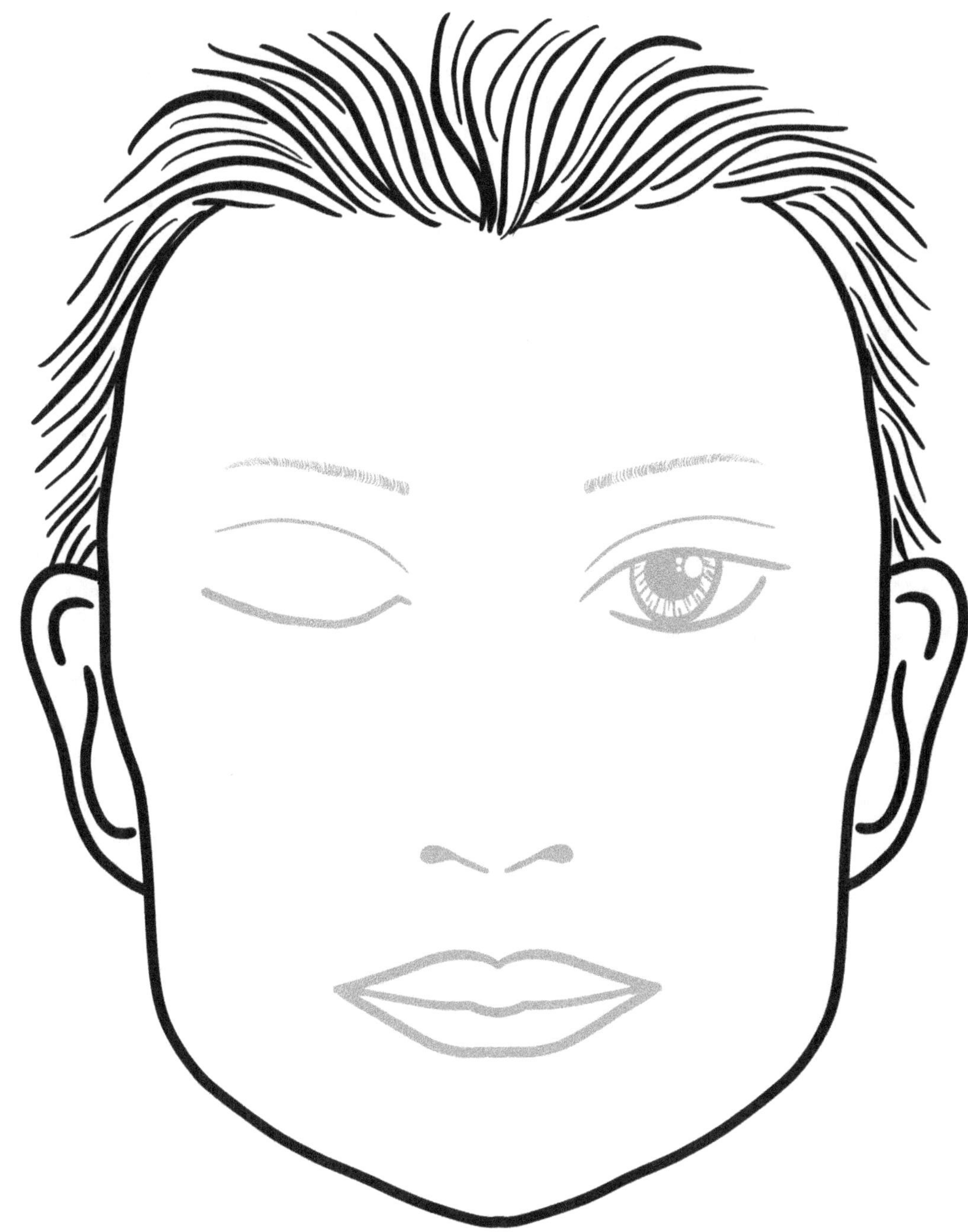

Details

Skin Tone _______________________

Eye Color _______________________

Hair Color _______________________

Lips (color, brand, etc.)

Lip Liner _______________________

Lip Color _______________________

Gloss _______________________

Eyes (color, brand, etc.)

Brows _______________________

Lid Color 1 _______________________

Lid Color 2 _______________________

Lid Color 3 _______________________

Crease _______________________

Eye Liner _______________________

Mascara _______________________

Face (color, brand, etc.)

Concealer _______________________

Foundation _______________________

Contour _______________________

Blush _______________________

Highlights _______________________

Powder _______________________

| Concealer | Foundation | Contour | Blush | Highlights | Powder | Eye Liner | Mascara |
| Brows | Lid Color 1 | Lid Color 2 | Lid Color 3 | Crease | Lip Liner | Lip Color | Lip Gloss |

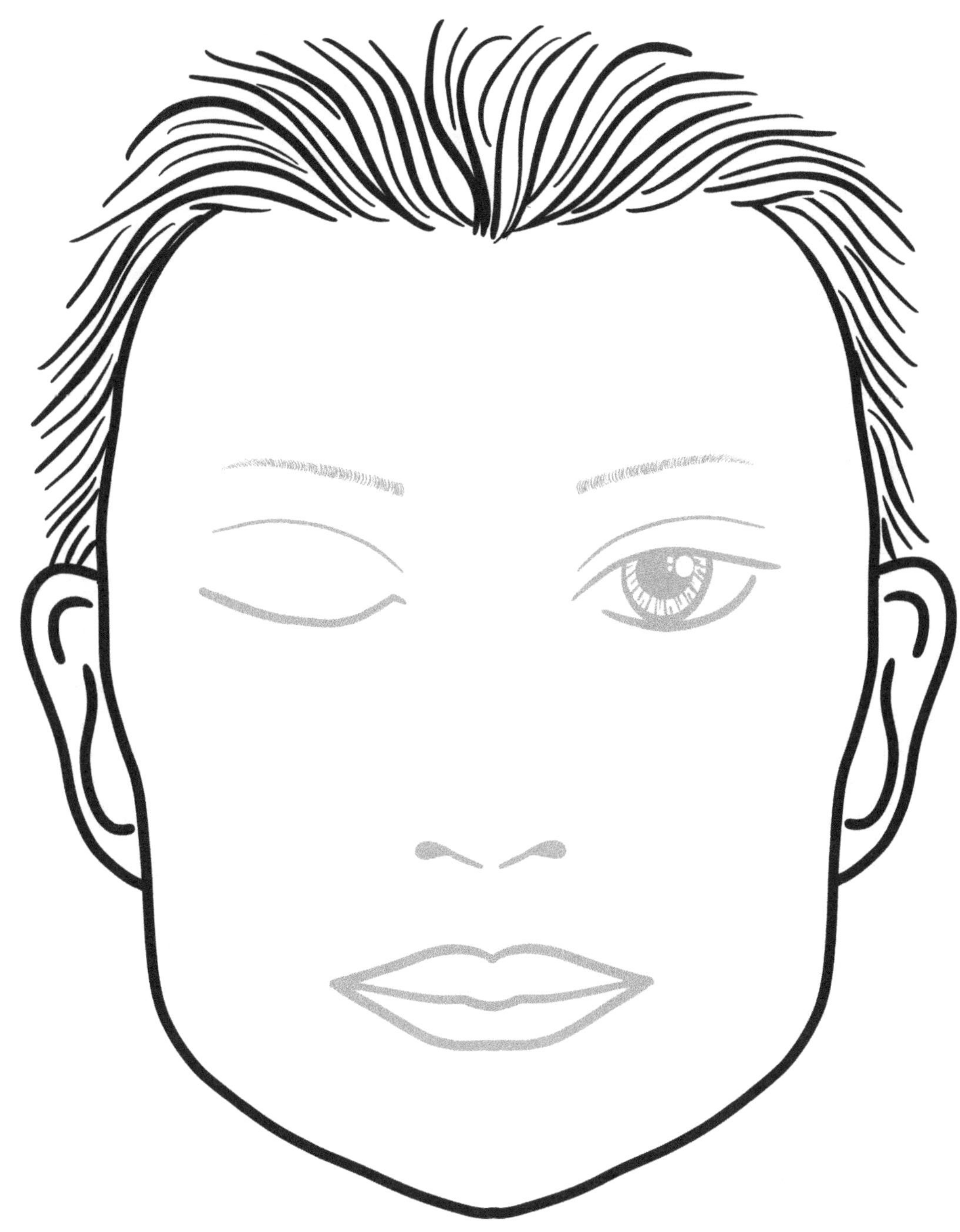

Details

Skin Tone __________________

Eye Color __________________

Hair Color __________________

Lips (color, brand, etc.)

Lip Liner __________________

Lip Color __________________

Gloss __________________

Eyes (color, brand, etc.)

Brows __________________

Lid Color 1 __________________

Lid Color 2 __________________

Lid Color 3 __________________

Crease __________________

Eye Liner __________________

Mascara __________________

Face (color, brand, etc.)

Concealer __________________

Foundation __________________

Contour __________________

Blush __________________

Highlights __________________

Powder __________________

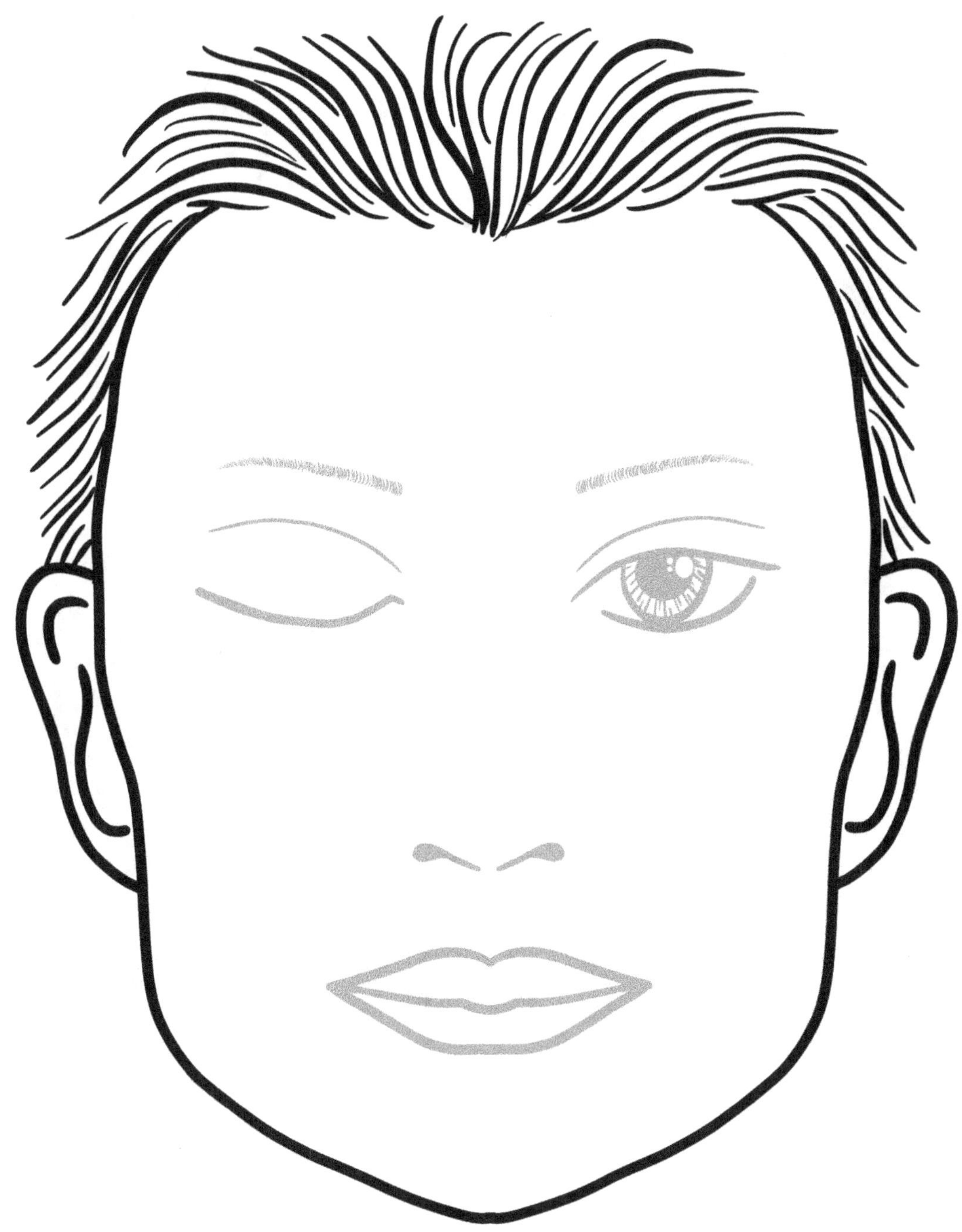

Date _______

Design/Client Name _______

Mascara	Lip Gloss
Eye Liner	Lip Color
Powder	Lip Liner
Highlights	Crease
Blush	Lid Color 3
Contour	Lid Color 2
Foundation	Lid Color 1
Concealer	Brows

Details

Skin Tone _______________________

Eye Color _______________________

Hair Color _______________________

Lips (color, brand, etc.)

Lip Liner _______________________

Lip Color _______________________

Gloss _______________________

Eyes (color, brand, etc.)

Brows _______________________

Lid Color 1 _______________________

Lid Color 2 _______________________

Lid Color 3 _______________________

Crease _______________________

Eye Liner _______________________

Mascara _______________________

Face (color, brand, etc.)

Concealer _______________________

Foundation _______________________

Contour _______________________

Blush _______________________

Highlights _______________________

Powder _______________________

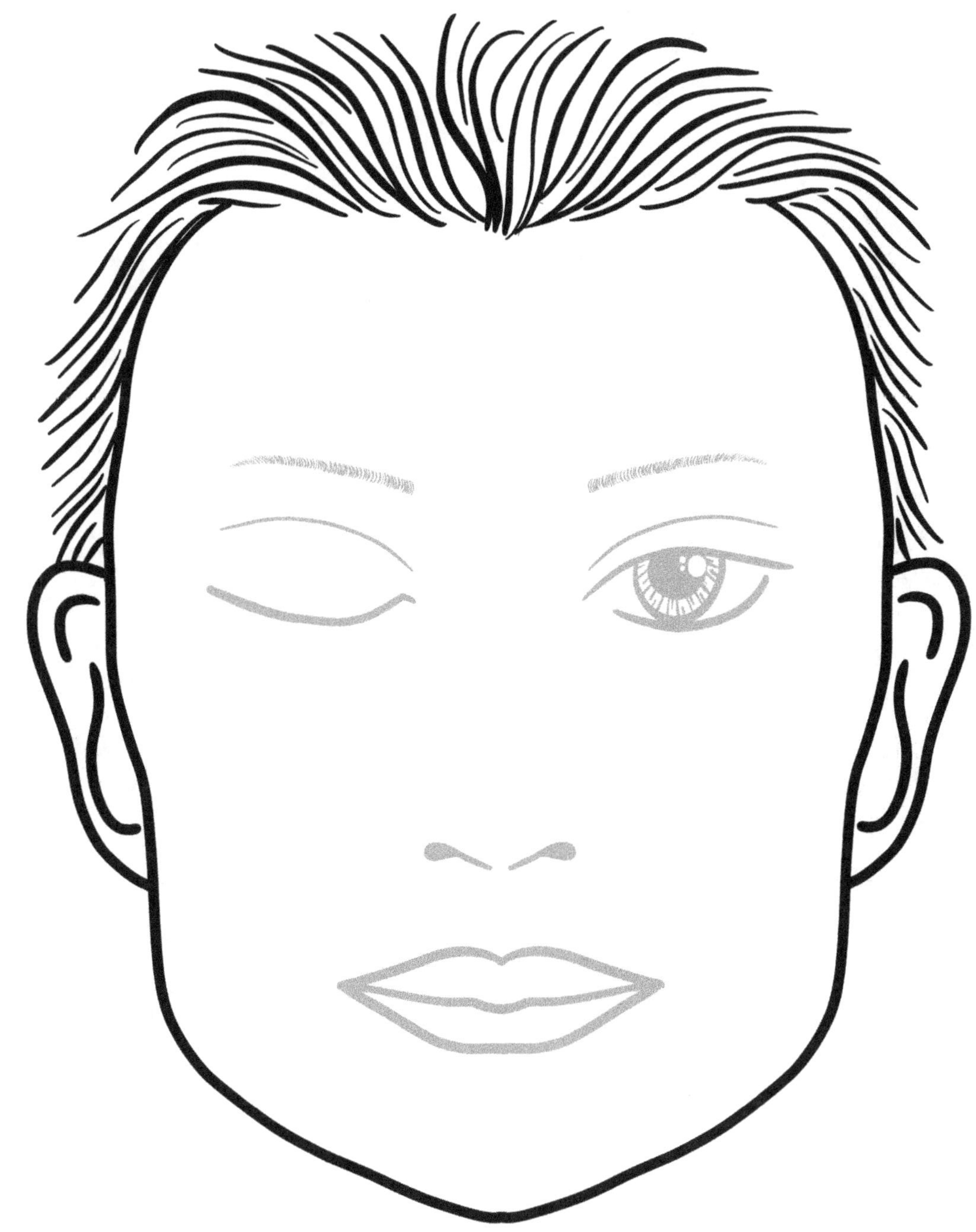

Details

Skin Tone _____________________

Eye Color _____________________

Hair Color _____________________

Lips (color, brand, etc.)

Lip Liner _____________________

Lip Color _____________________

Gloss _____________________

Eyes (color, brand, etc.)

Brows _____________________

Lid Color 1 _____________________

Lid Color 2 _____________________

Lid Color 3 _____________________

Crease _____________________

Eye Liner _____________________

Mascara _____________________

Face (color, brand, etc.)

Concealer _____________________

Foundation _____________________

Contour _____________________

Blush _____________________

Highlights _____________________

Powder _____________________

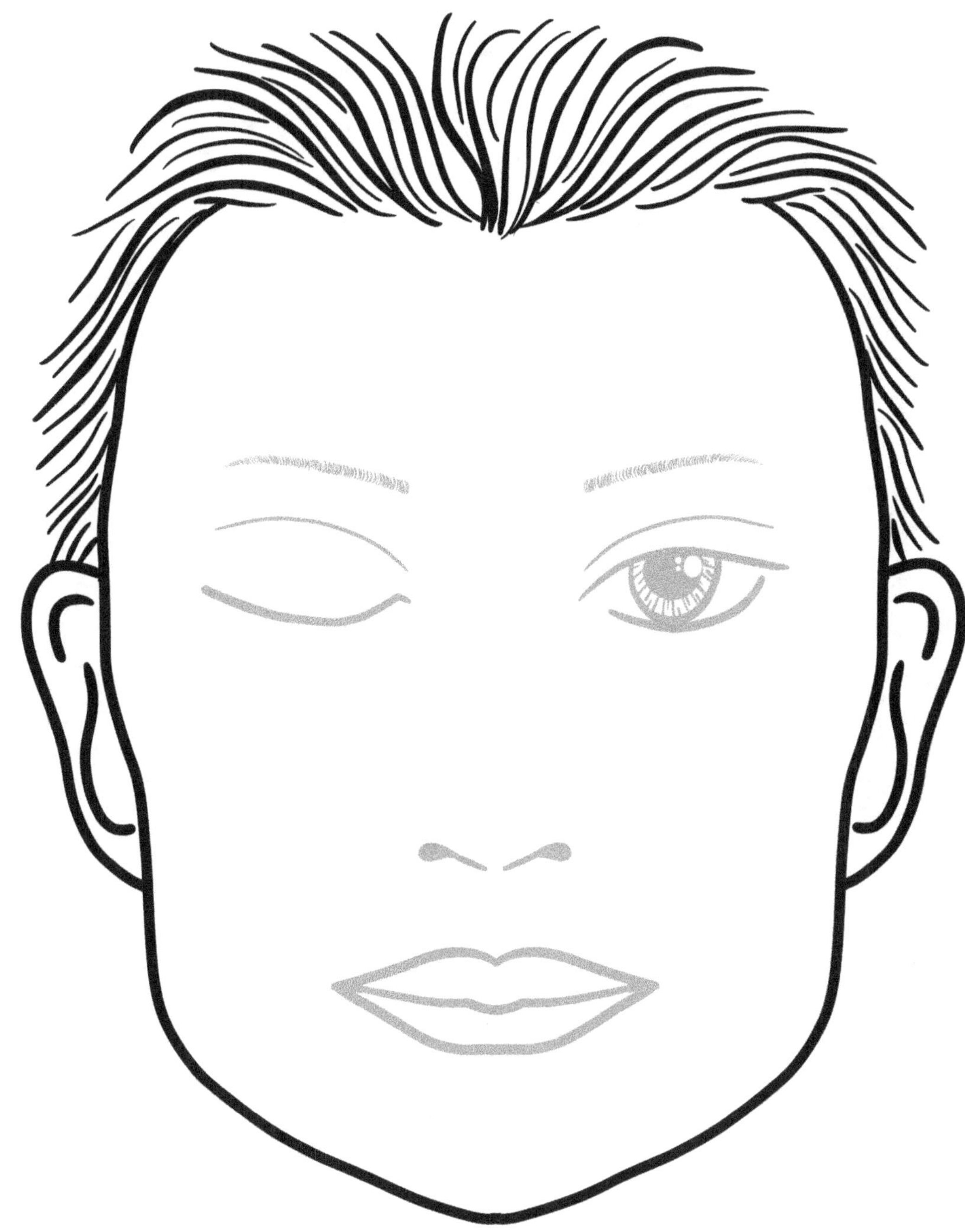

Date ______

Design/Client Name ______

Concealer	Foundation	Contour	Blush	Highlights	Powder	Eye Liner	Mascara
	Lid Color 1	Lid Color 2	Lid Color 3	Crease	Lip Liner	Lip Color	Lip Gloss
	Brows						

Details

Skin Tone ______

Eye Color ______

Hair Color ______

Lips (color, brand, etc.)

Lip Liner ______

Lip Color ______

Gloss ______

Eyes (color, brand, etc.)

Brows ______

Lid Color 1 ______

Lid Color 2 ______

Lid Color 3 ______

Crease ______

Eye Liner ______

Mascara ______

Face (color, brand, etc.)

Concealer ______

Foundation ______

Contour ______

Blush ______

Highlights ______

Powder ______

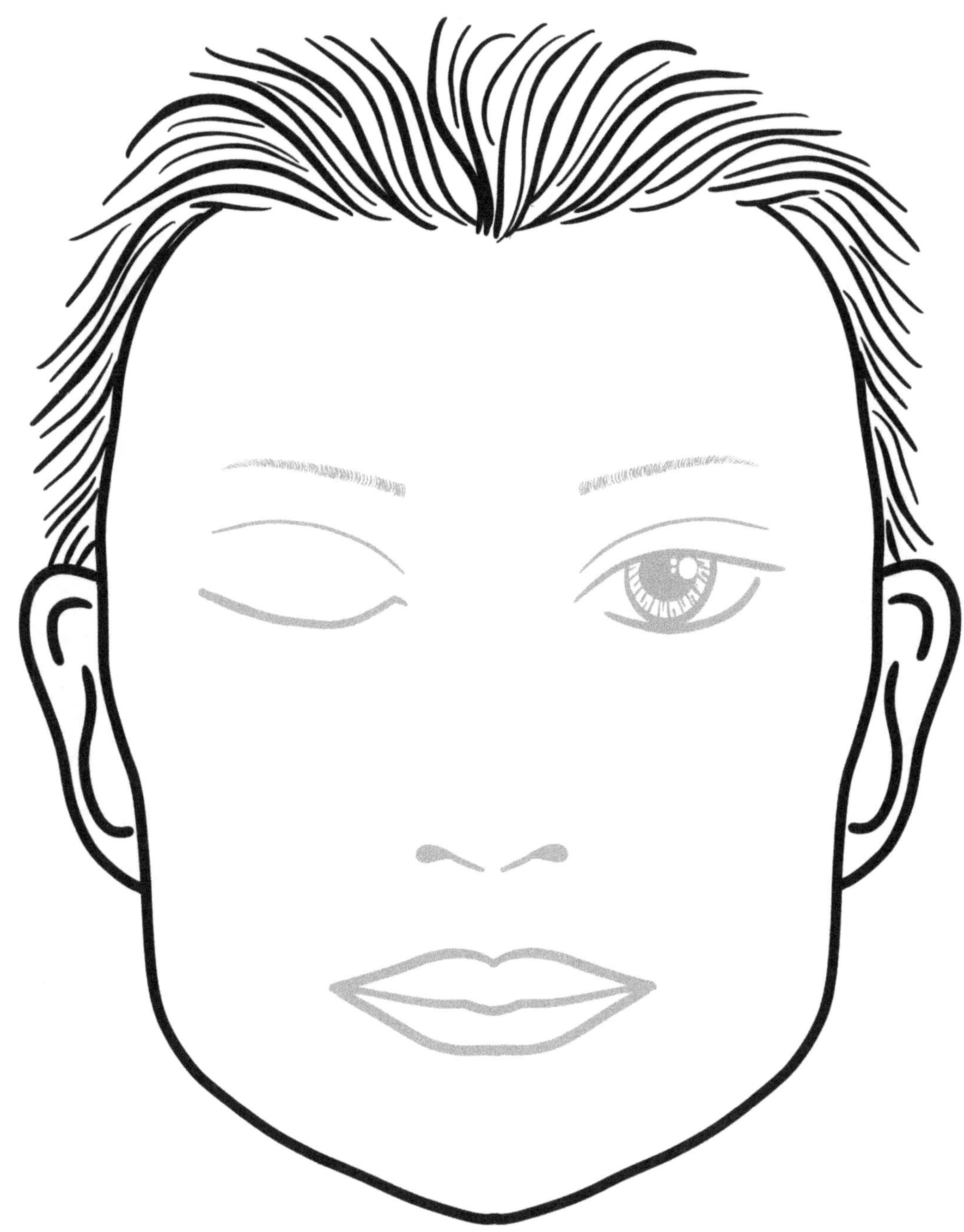

Details

Skin Tone _______________________

Eye Color _______________________

Hair Color _______________________

Lips (color, brand, etc.)

Lip Liner _______________________

Lip Color _______________________

Gloss _______________________

Eyes (color, brand, etc.)

Brows _______________________

Lid Color 1 _______________________

Lid Color 2 _______________________

Lid Color 3 _______________________

Crease _______________________

Eye Liner _______________________

Mascara _______________________

Face (color, brand, etc.)

Concealer _______________________

Foundation _______________________

Contour _______________________

Blush _______________________

Highlights _______________________

Powder _______________________

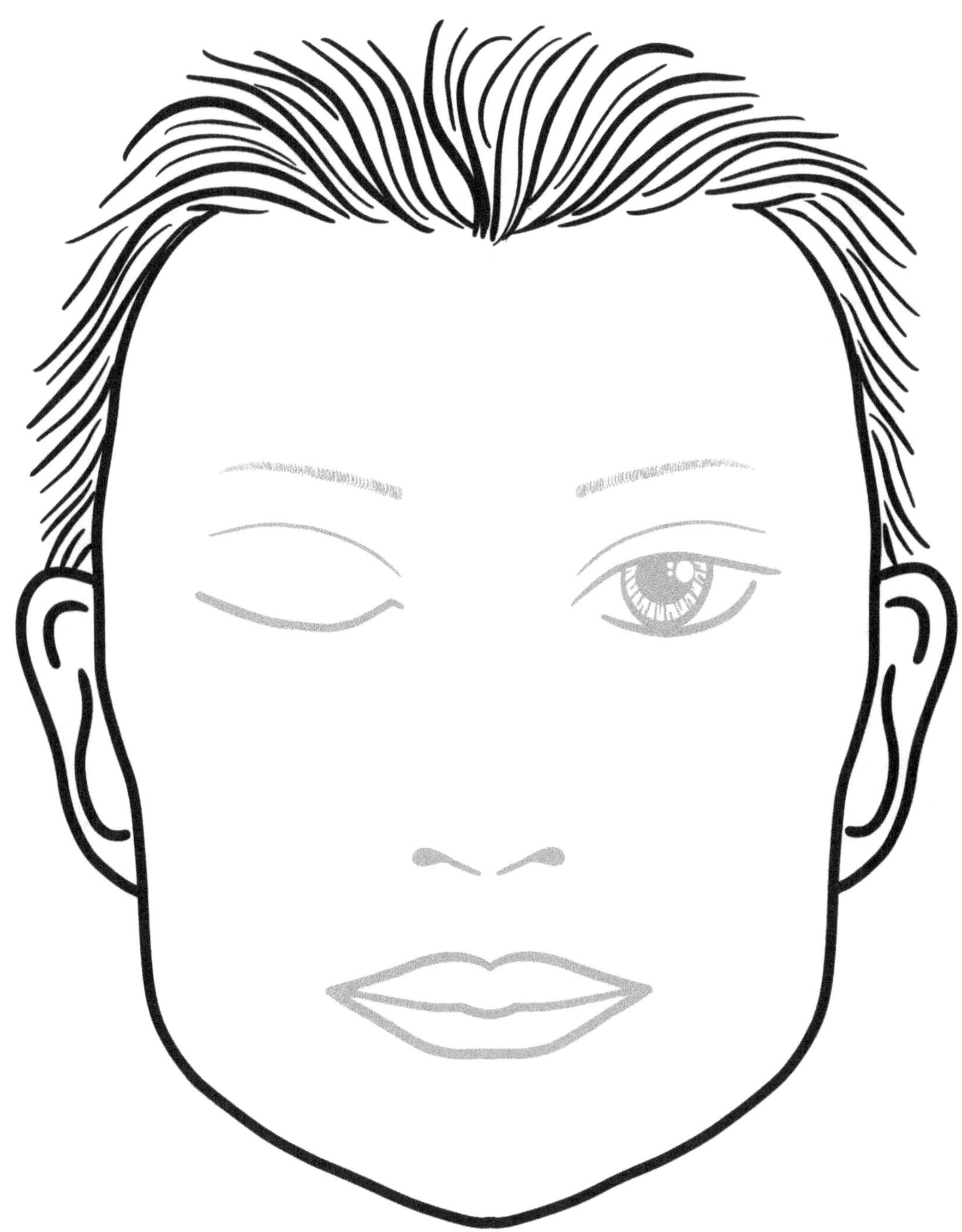

Details

Skin Tone _________________

Eye Color _________________

Hair Color _________________

Lips (color, brand, etc.)

Lip Liner _________________

Lip Color _________________

Gloss _________________

Eyes (color, brand, etc.)

Brows _________________

Lid Color 1 _________________

Lid Color 2 _________________

Lid Color 3 _________________

Crease _________________

Eye Liner _________________

Mascara _________________

Face (color, brand, etc.)

Concealer _________________

Foundation _________________

Contour _________________

Blush _________________

Highlights _________________

Powder _________________

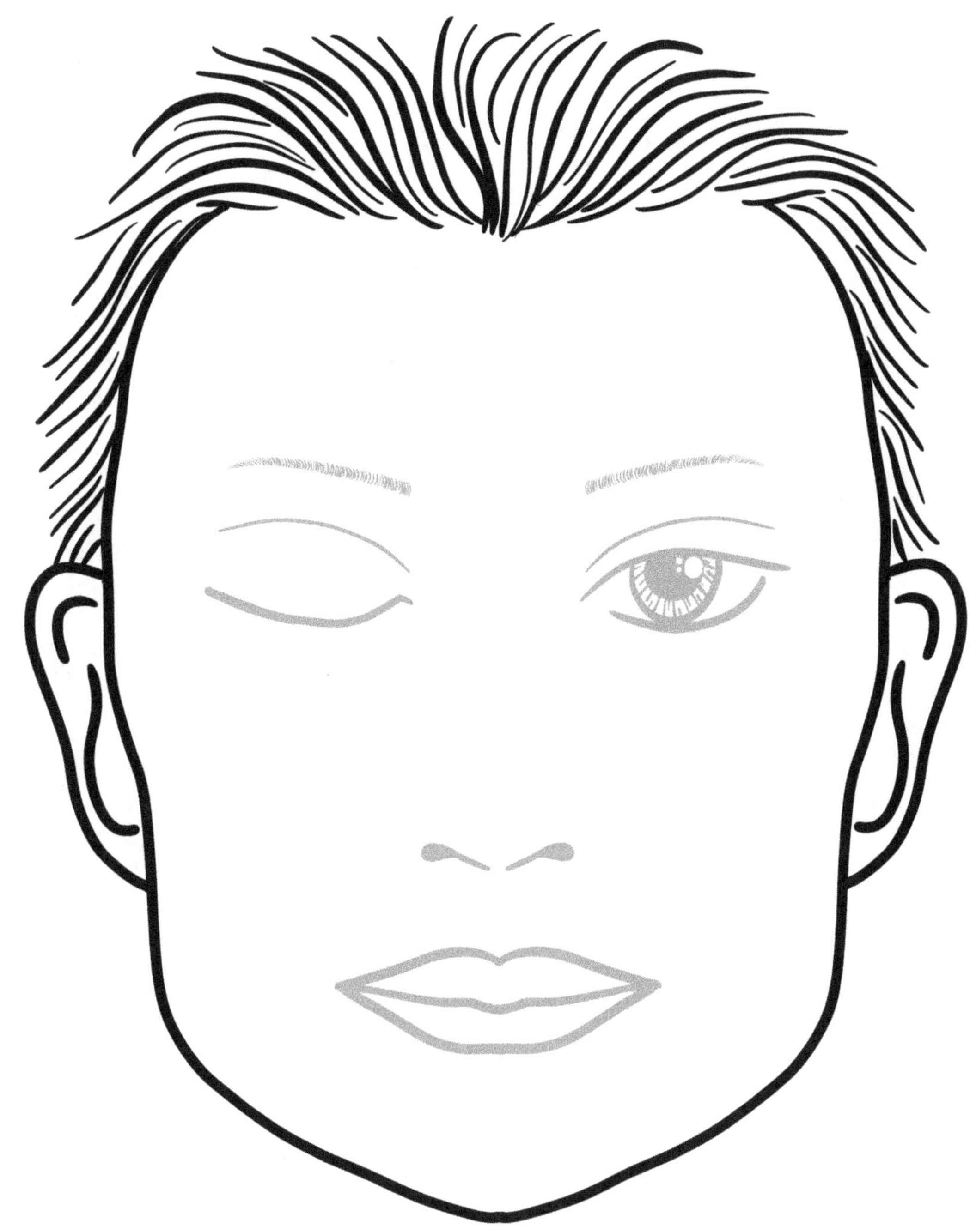

<table>
<tr><td>Date</td><td>Mascara</td><td>Lip Gloss</td></tr>
<tr><td></td><td>Eye Liner</td><td>Lip Color</td></tr>
<tr><td></td><td>Powder</td><td>Lip Liner</td></tr>
<tr><td></td><td>Highlights</td><td>Crease</td></tr>
<tr><td></td><td>Blush</td><td>Lid Color 3</td></tr>
<tr><td></td><td>Contour</td><td>Lid Color 2</td></tr>
<tr><td></td><td>Foundation</td><td>Lid Color 1</td></tr>
<tr><td>Design/Client Name</td><td>Concealer</td><td>Brows</td></tr>
</table>

Details

Skin Tone _______________________

Eye Color _______________________

Hair Color _______________________

Lips (color, brand, etc.)

Lip Liner _______________________

Lip Color _______________________

Gloss _______________________

Eyes (color, brand, etc.)

Brows _______________________

Lid Color 1 _______________________

Lid Color 2 _______________________

Lid Color 3 _______________________

Crease _______________________

Eye Liner _______________________

Mascara _______________________

Face (color, brand, etc.)

Concealer _______________________

Foundation _______________________

Contour _______________________

Blush _______________________

Highlights _______________________

Powder _______________________

Concealer	Foundation	Contour	Blush	Highlights	Powder	Eye Liner	Mascara
Brows	Lid Color 1	Lid Color 2	Lid Color 3	Crease	Lip Liner	Lip Color	Lip Gloss

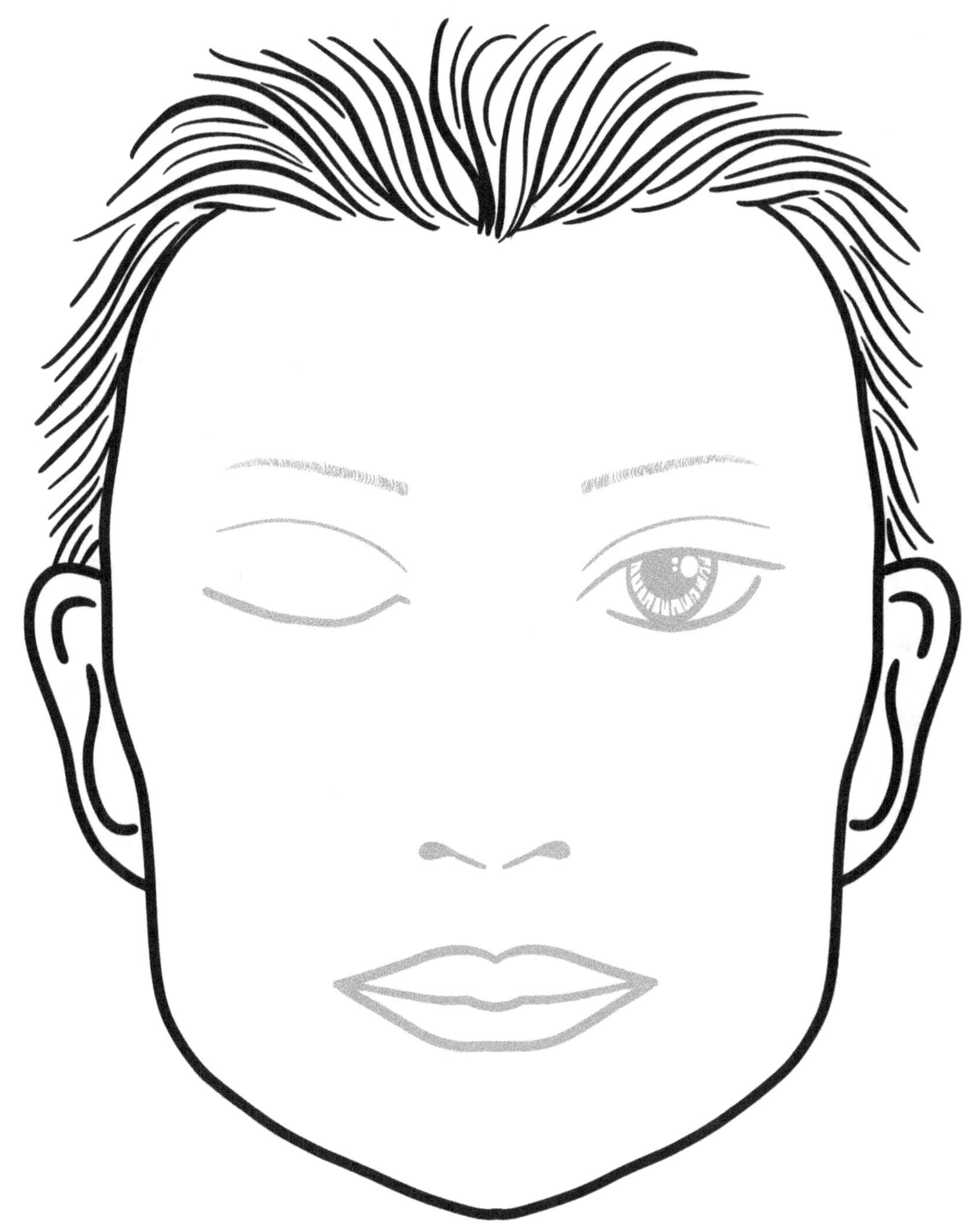

Details

Skin Tone _______________________

Eye Color _______________________

Hair Color _______________________

Lips (color, brand, etc.)

Lip Liner _______________________

Lip Color _______________________

Gloss _______________________

Eyes (color, brand, etc.)

Brows _______________________

Lid Color 1 _______________________

Lid Color 2 _______________________

Lid Color 3 _______________________

Crease _______________________

Eye Liner _______________________

Mascara _______________________

Face (color, brand, etc.)

Concealer _______________________

Foundation _______________________

Contour _______________________

Blush _______________________

Highlights _______________________

Powder _______________________

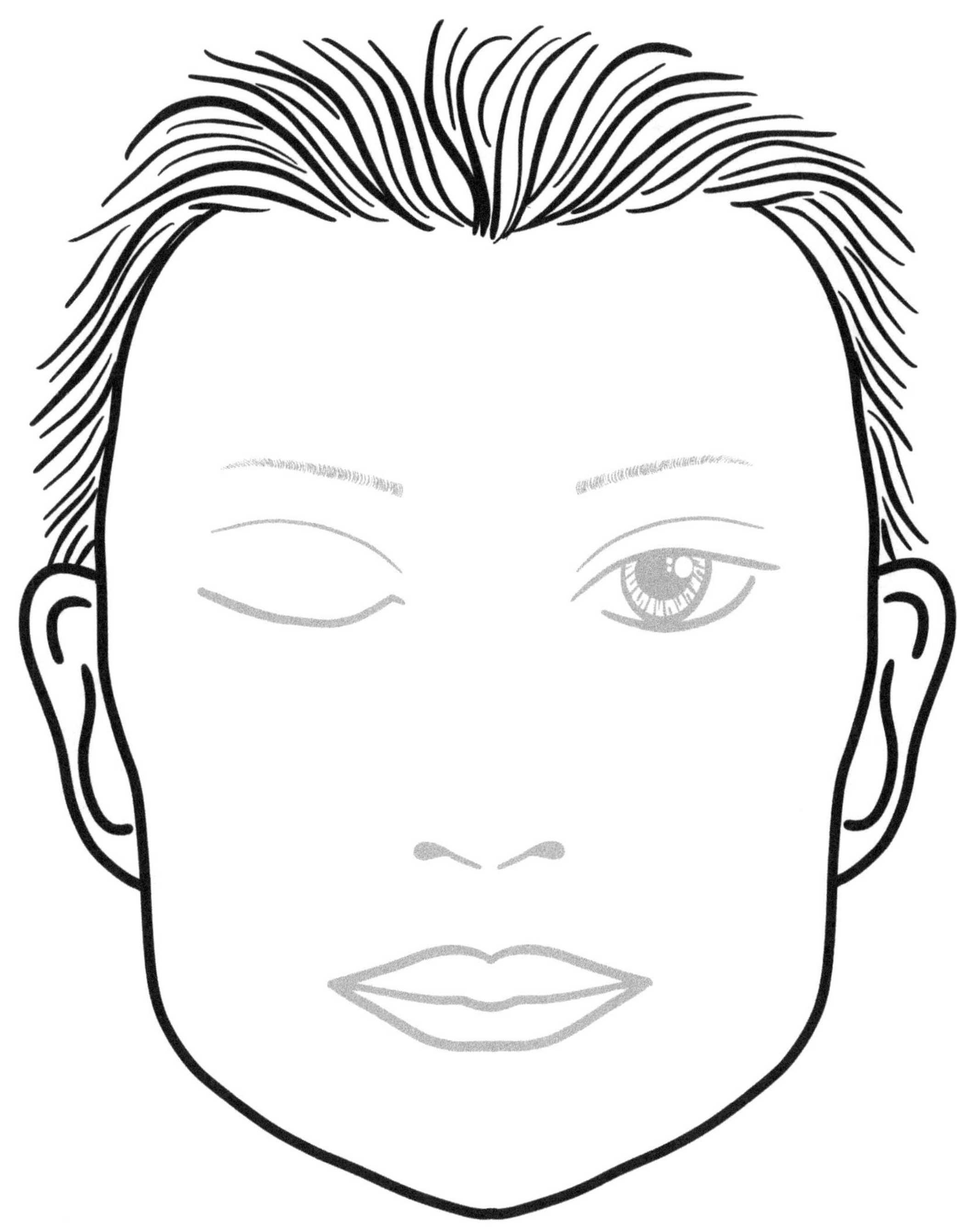

Details

Skin Tone _______________________

Eye Color _______________________

Hair Color _______________________

Lips (color, brand, etc.)

Lip Liner _______________________

Lip Color _______________________

Gloss _______________________

Eyes (color, brand, etc.)

Brows _______________________

Lid Color 1 _______________________

Lid Color 2 _______________________

Lid Color 3 _______________________

Crease _______________________

Eye Liner _______________________

Mascara _______________________

Face (color, brand, etc.)

Concealer _______________________

Foundation _______________________

Contour _______________________

Blush _______________________

Highlights _______________________

Powder _______________________

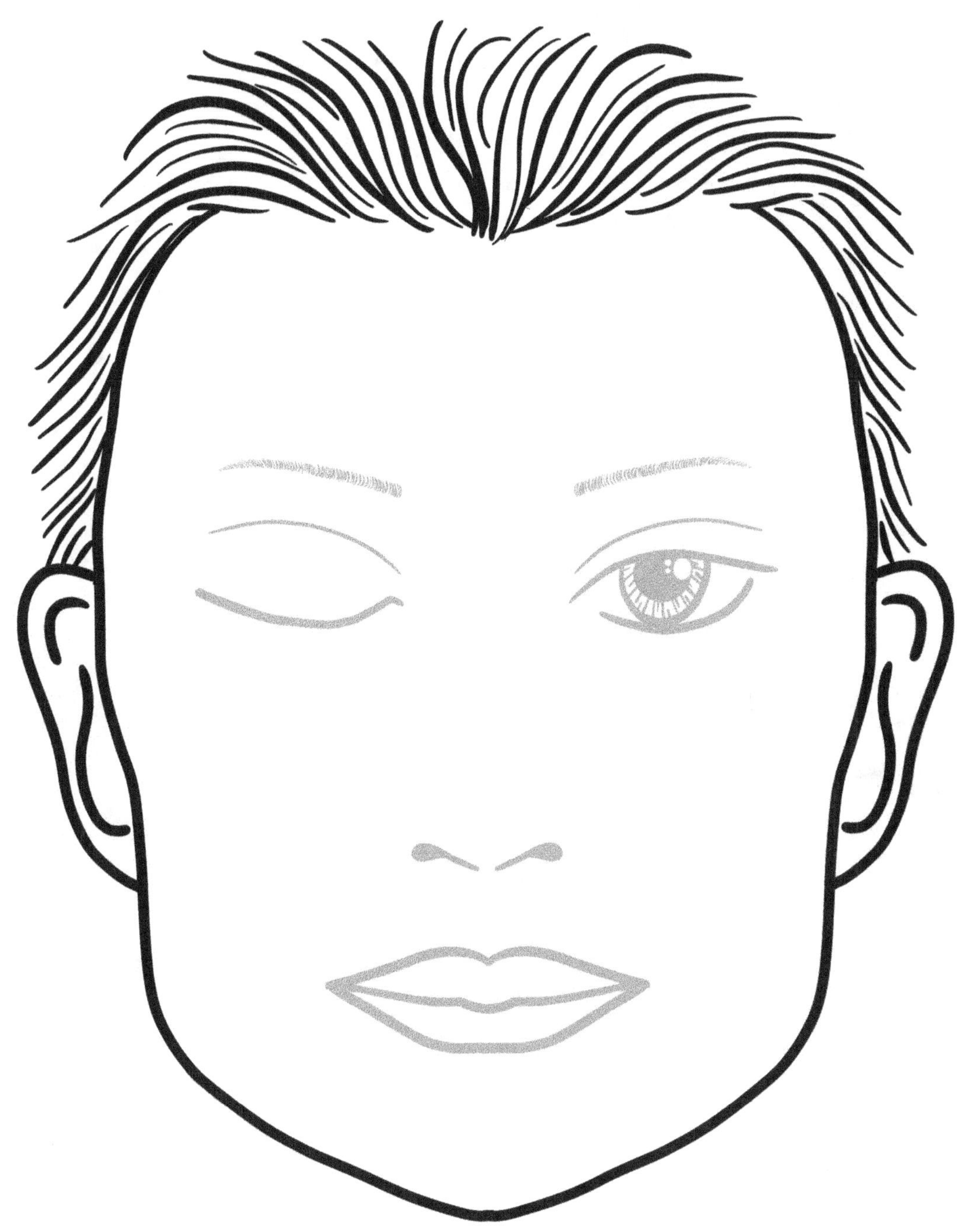

Details

Skin Tone _______________________

Eye Color _______________________

Hair Color _______________________

Lips (color, brand, etc.)

Lip Liner _______________________

Lip Color _______________________

Gloss _______________________

Eyes (color, brand, etc.)

Brows _______________________

Lid Color 1 _______________________

Lid Color 2 _______________________

Lid Color 3 _______________________

Crease _______________________

Eye Liner _______________________

Mascara _______________________

Face (color, brand, etc.)

Concealer _______________________

Foundation _______________________

Contour _______________________

Blush _______________________

Highlights _______________________

Powder _______________________

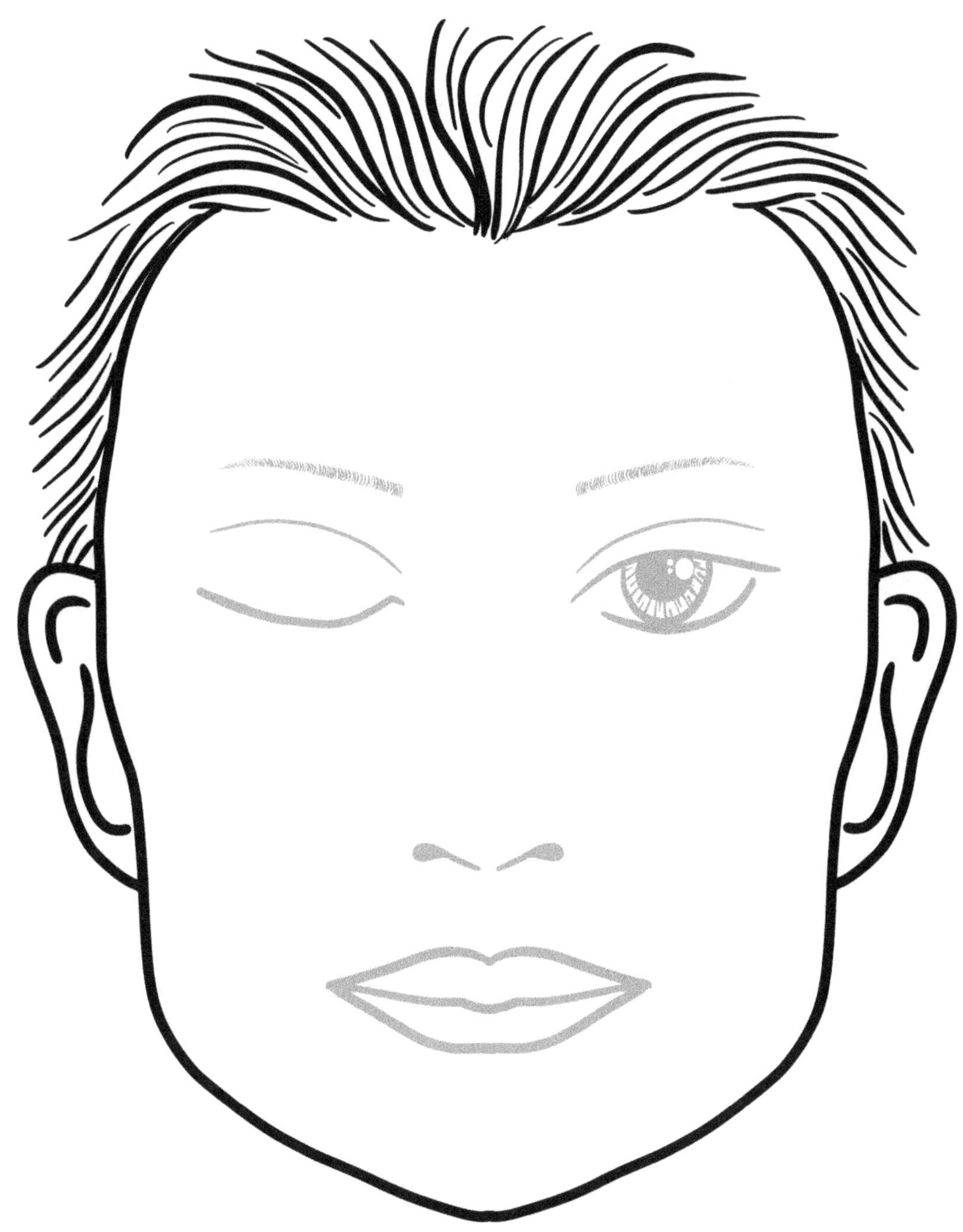

Details

Skin Tone ___________________

Eye Color ___________________

Hair Color ___________________

Lips (color, brand, etc.)

Lip Liner ___________________

Lip Color ___________________

Gloss ___________________

Eyes (color, brand, etc.)

Brows ___________________

Lid Color 1 ___________________

Lid Color 2 ___________________

Lid Color 3 ___________________

Crease ___________________

Eye Liner ___________________

Mascara ___________________

Face (color, brand, etc.)

Concealer ___________________

Foundation ___________________

Contour ___________________

Blush ___________________

Highlights ___________________

Powder ___________________

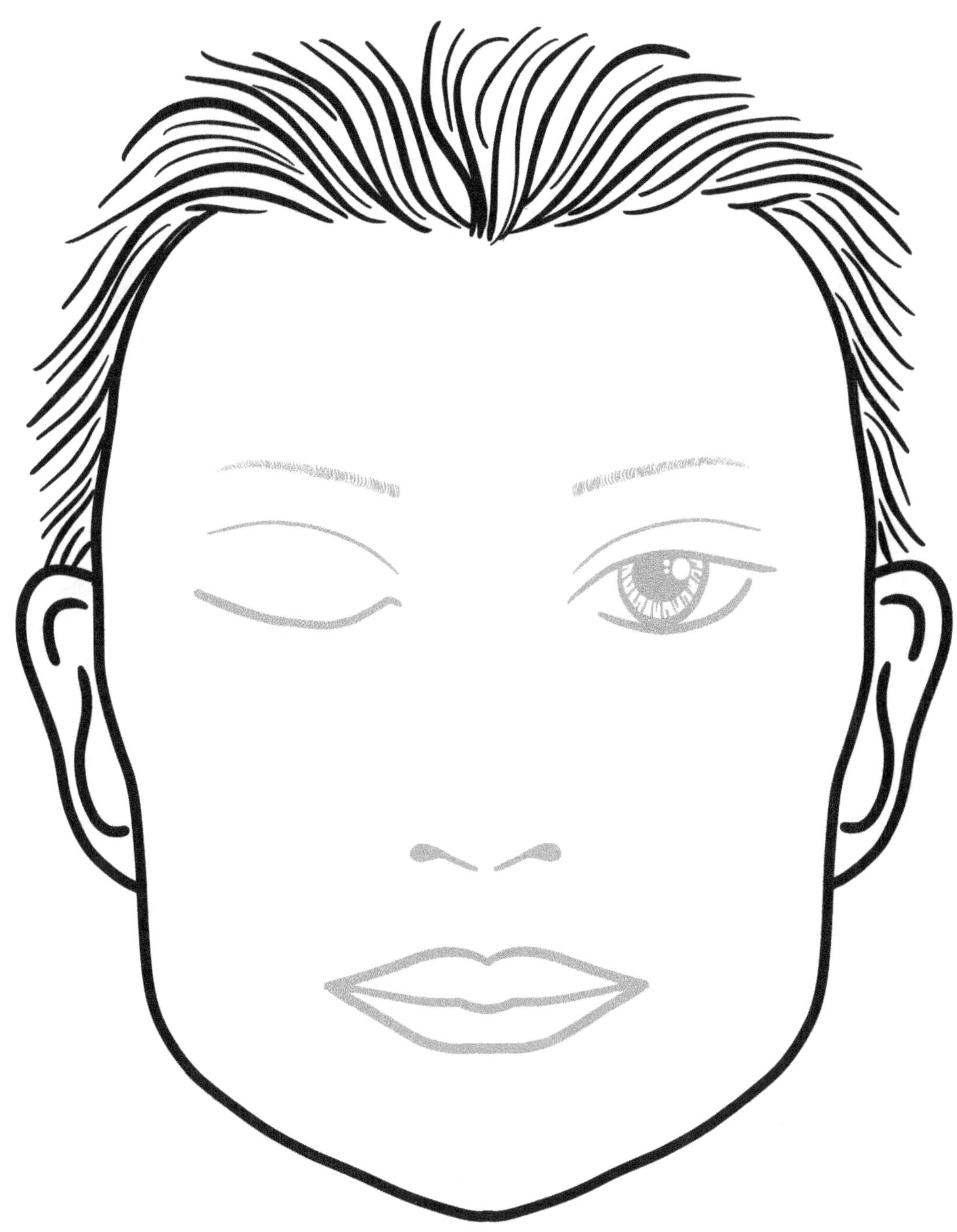

Date		Design/Client Name
Mascara	Eye Liner	Powder	Highlights	Blush	Contour	Foundation	Concealer
Lip Gloss	Lip Color	Lip Liner	Crease	Lid Color 3	Lid Color 2	Lid Color 1	Brows

Details

Skin Tone _______________________

Eye Color _______________________

Hair Color _______________________

Lips (color, brand, etc.)

Lip Liner _______________________

Lip Color _______________________

Gloss _______________________

Eyes (color, brand, etc.)

Brows _______________________

Lid Color 1 _______________________

Lid Color 2 _______________________

Lid Color 3 _______________________

Crease _______________________

Eye Liner _______________________

Mascara _______________________

Face (color, brand, etc.)

Concealer _______________________

Foundation _______________________

Contour _______________________

Blush _______________________

Highlights _______________________

Powder _______________________

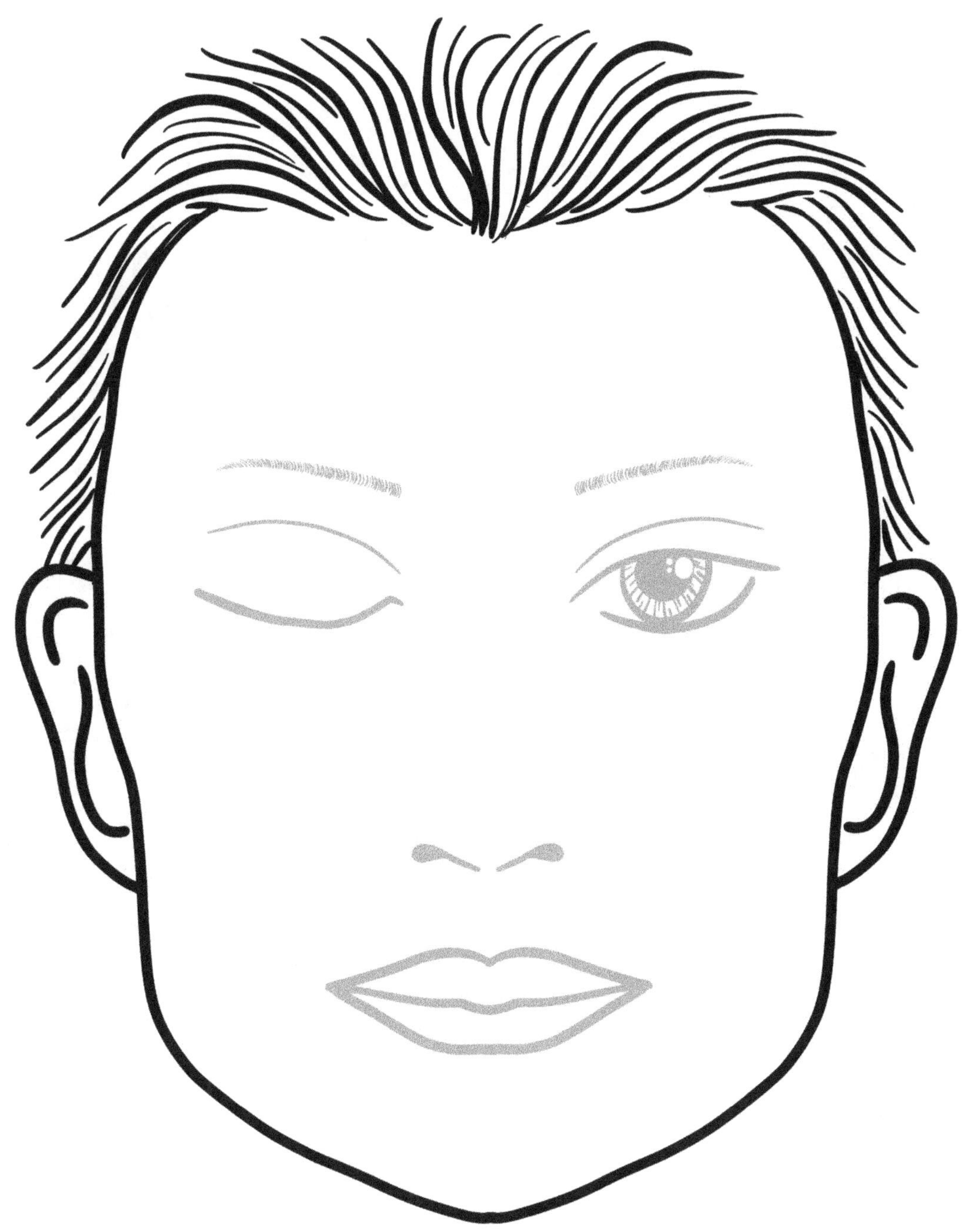

Details

Skin Tone______________________

Eye Color ______________________

Hair Color______________________

Lips (color, brand, etc.)

Lip Liner ______________________

Lip Color ______________________

Gloss ______________________

Eyes (color, brand, etc.)

Brows ______________________

Lid Color 1 ______________________

Lid Color 2 ______________________

Lid Color 3 ______________________

Crease______________________

Eye Liner______________________

Mascara______________________

Face (color, brand, etc.)

Concealer______________________

Foundation______________________

Contour______________________

Blush ______________________

Highlights ______________________

Powder______________________

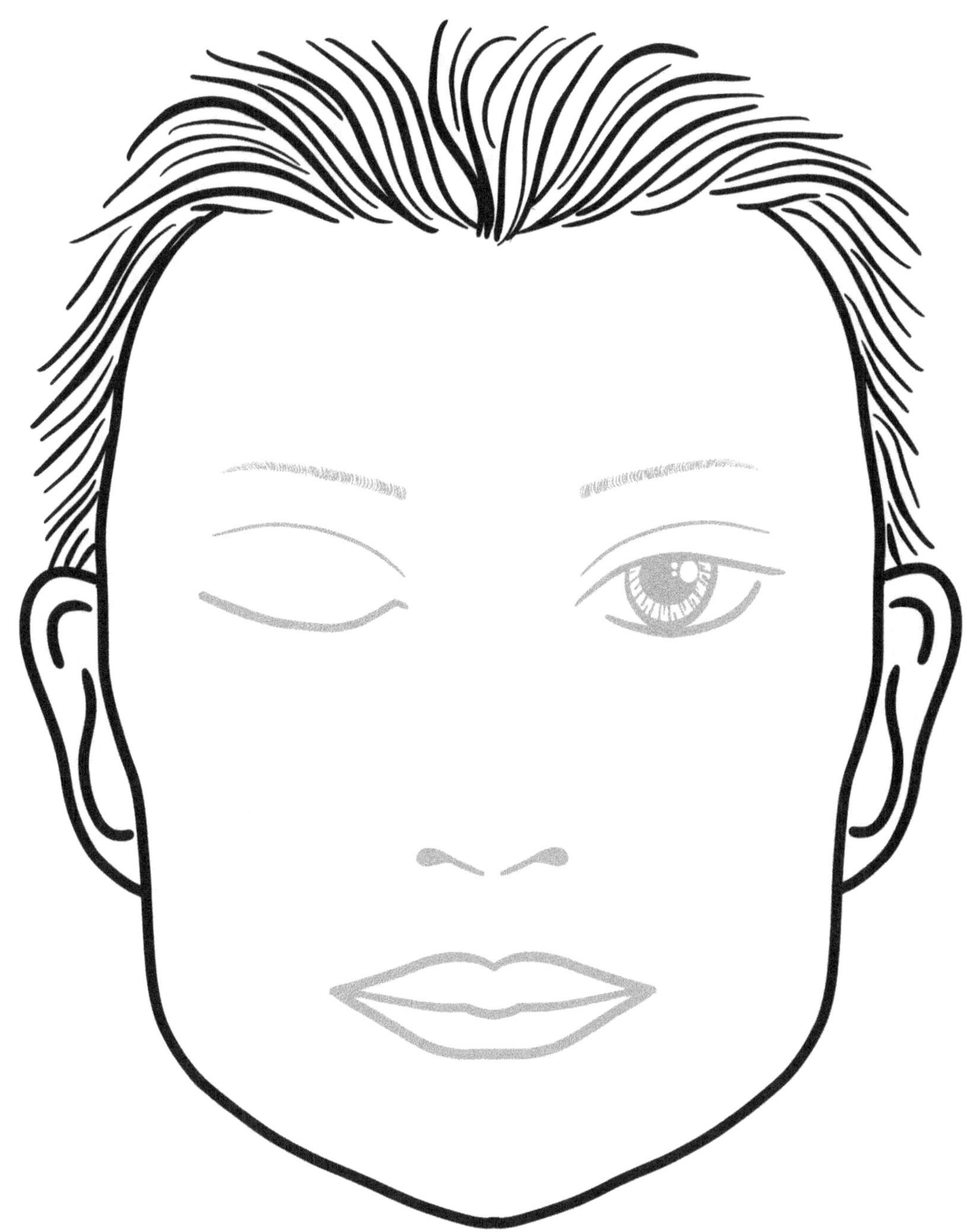

Date

Design/Client Name

Concealer	Foundation	Contour	Blush	Highlights	Powder	Eye Liner	Mascara
Brows	Lid Color 1	Lid Color 2	Lid Color 3	Crease	Lip Liner	Lip Color	Lip Gloss

Details

Skin Tone _______________________

Eye Color _______________________

Hair Color _______________________

Lips (color, brand, etc.)

Lip Liner _______________________

Lip Color _______________________

Gloss _______________________

Eyes (color, brand, etc.)

Brows _______________________

Lid Color 1 _______________________

Lid Color 2 _______________________

Lid Color 3 _______________________

Crease _______________________

Eye Liner _______________________

Mascara _______________________

Face (color, brand, etc.)

Concealer _______________________

Foundation _______________________

Contour _______________________

Blush _______________________

Highlights _______________________

Powder _______________________

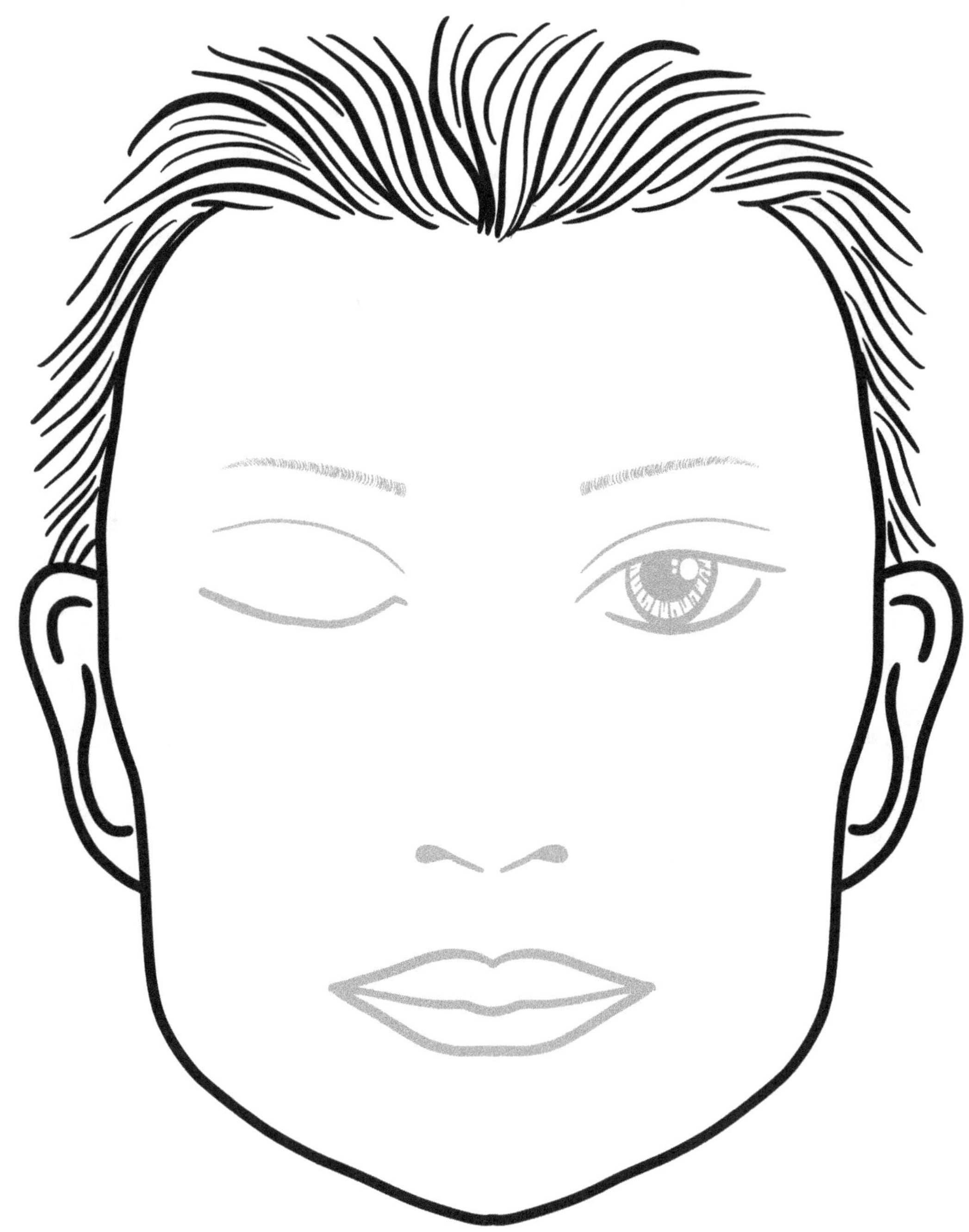

Design/Client Name _______________

Date _______________

Concealer	Foundation	Contour	Blush	Highlights	Powder	Eye Liner	Mascara
Brows	Lid Color 1	Lid Color 2	Lid Color 3	Crease	Lip Liner	Lip Color	Lip Gloss

Details

Skin Tone _______________

Eye Color _______________

Hair Color _______________

Lips (color, brand, etc.)

Lip Liner _______________

Lip Color _______________

Gloss _______________

Eyes (color, brand, etc.)

Brows _______________

Lid Color 1 _______________

Lid Color 2 _______________

Lid Color 3 _______________

Crease _______________

Eye Liner _______________

Mascara _______________

Face (color, brand, etc.)

Concealer _______________

Foundation _______________

Contour _______________

Blush _______________

Highlights _______________

Powder _______________

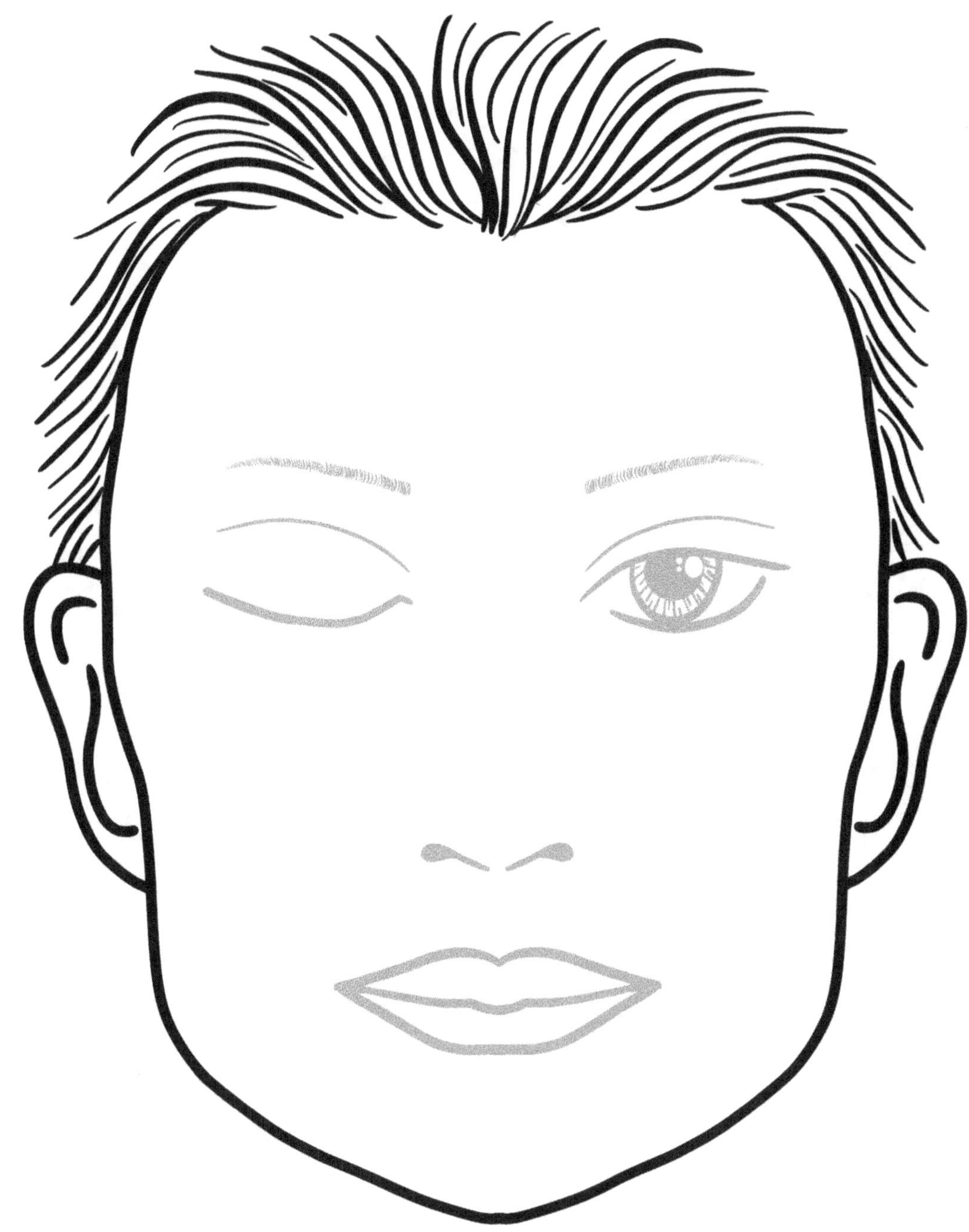

Date _______

Design/Client Name _______

Concealer	Foundation	Contour	Blush	Highlights	Powder	Eye Liner	Mascara
Brows	Lid Color 1	Lid Color 2	Lid Color 3	Crease	Lip Liner	Lip Color	Lip Gloss

Details

Skin Tone _____________________

Eye Color _____________________

Hair Color _____________________

Lips (color, brand, etc.)

Lip Liner _____________________

Lip Color _____________________

Gloss _____________________

Eyes (color, brand, etc.)

Brows _____________________

Lid Color 1 _____________________

Lid Color 2 _____________________

Lid Color 3 _____________________

Crease _____________________

Eye Liner _____________________

Mascara _____________________

Face (color, brand, etc.)

Concealer _____________________

Foundation _____________________

Contour _____________________

Blush _____________________

Highlights _____________________

Powder _____________________

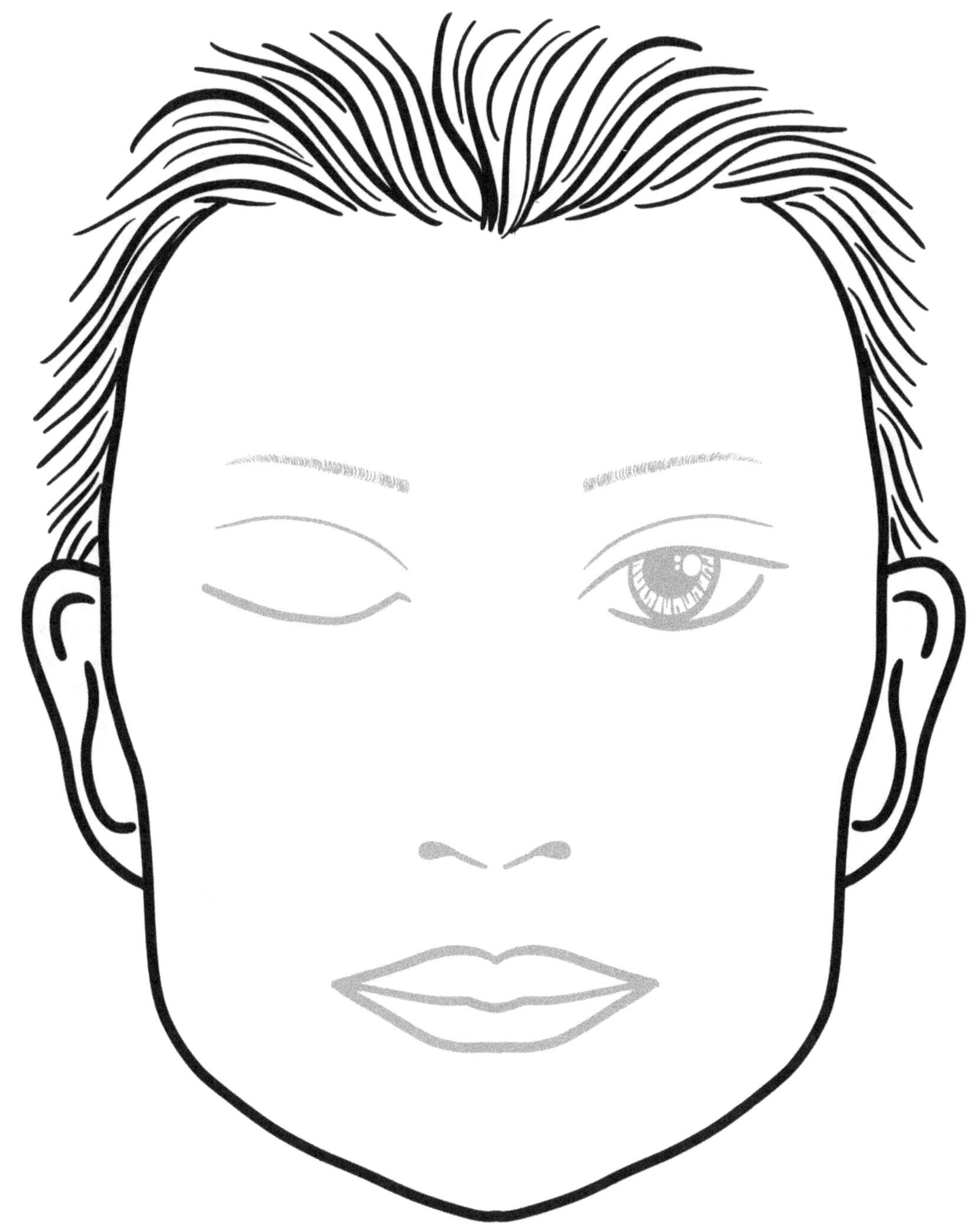

| Concealer | Foundation | Contour | Blush | Highlights | Powder | Eye Liner | Mascara |
| Brows | Lid Color 1 | Lid Color 2 | Lid Color 3 | Crease | Lip Liner | Lip Color | Lip Gloss |

Details

Skin Tone________________

Eye Color ________________

Hair Color________________

Lips (color, brand, etc.)

Lip Liner ________________

Lip Color ________________

Gloss ________________

Eyes (color, brand, etc.)

Brows ________________

Lid Color 1 ________________

Lid Color 2 ________________

Lid Color 3 ________________

Crease________________

Eye Liner________________

Mascara ________________

Face (color, brand, etc.)

Concealer________________

Foundation________________

Contour________________

Blush ________________

Highlights ________________

Powder________________

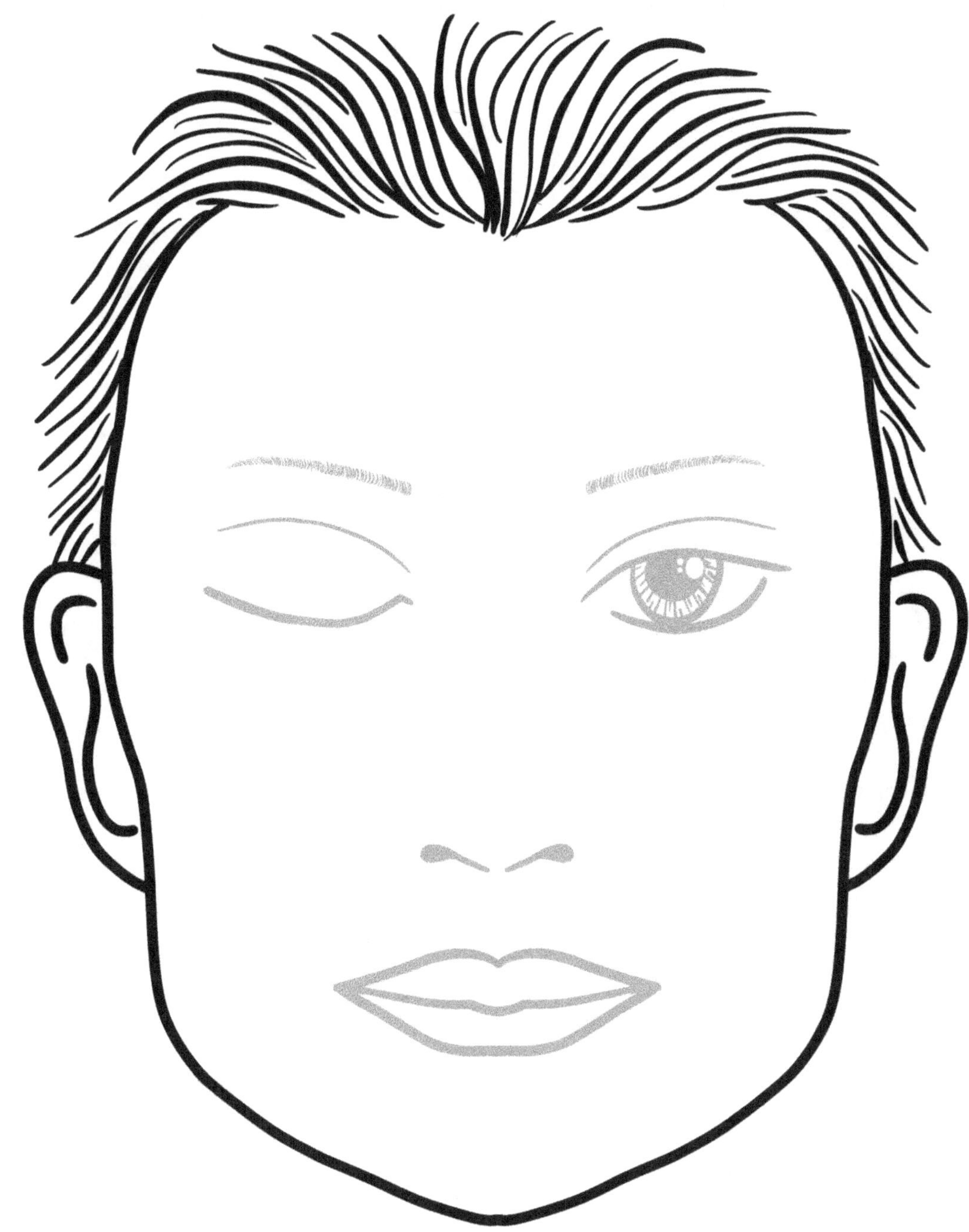

<table>
<tr><td>Date</td><td>Mascara</td><td>Eye Liner</td><td>Powder</td><td>Highlights</td><td>Blush</td><td>Contour</td><td>Foundation</td><td>Concealer</td></tr>
<tr><td></td><td>Lip Gloss</td><td>Lip Color</td><td>Lip Liner</td><td>Crease</td><td>Lid Color 3</td><td>Lid Color 2</td><td>Lid Color 1</td><td>Brows</td></tr>
</table>

Design/Client Name

Details

Skin Tone ___________________

Eye Color ___________________

Hair Color ___________________

Lips (color, brand, etc.)

Lip Liner ___________________

Lip Color ___________________

Gloss ___________________

Eyes (color, brand, etc.)

Brows ___________________

Lid Color 1 ___________________

Lid Color 2 ___________________

Lid Color 3 ___________________

Crease ___________________

Eye Liner ___________________

Mascara ___________________

Face (color, brand, etc.)

Concealer ___________________

Foundation ___________________

Contour ___________________

Blush ___________________

Highlights ___________________

Powder ___________________

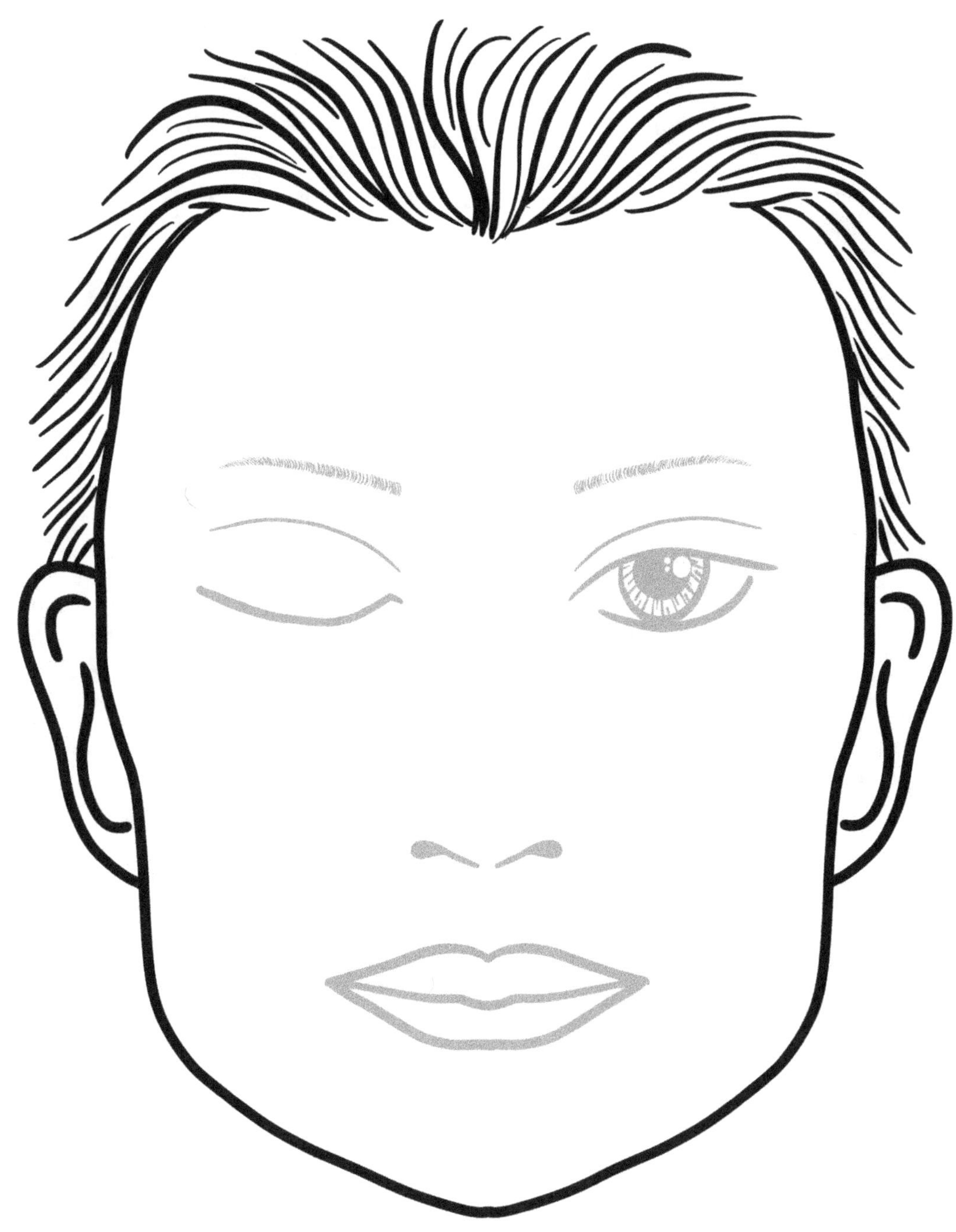

Date _______________

Design/Client Name _______________

Concealer	Foundation	Contour	Blush	Highlights	Powder	Eye Liner	Mascara
	Lid Color 1	Lid Color 2	Lid Color 3	Crease	Lip Liner	Lip Color	Lip Gloss
Brows							

Details

Skin Tone _______________

Eye Color _______________

Hair Color _______________

Lips (color, brand, etc.)

Lip Liner _______________

Lip Color _______________

Gloss _______________

Eyes (color, brand, etc.)

Brows _______________

Lid Color 1 _______________

Lid Color 2 _______________

Lid Color 3 _______________

Crease _______________

Eye Liner _______________

Mascara _______________

Face (color, brand, etc.)

Concealer _______________

Foundation _______________

Contour _______________

Blush _______________

Highlights _______________

Powder _______________

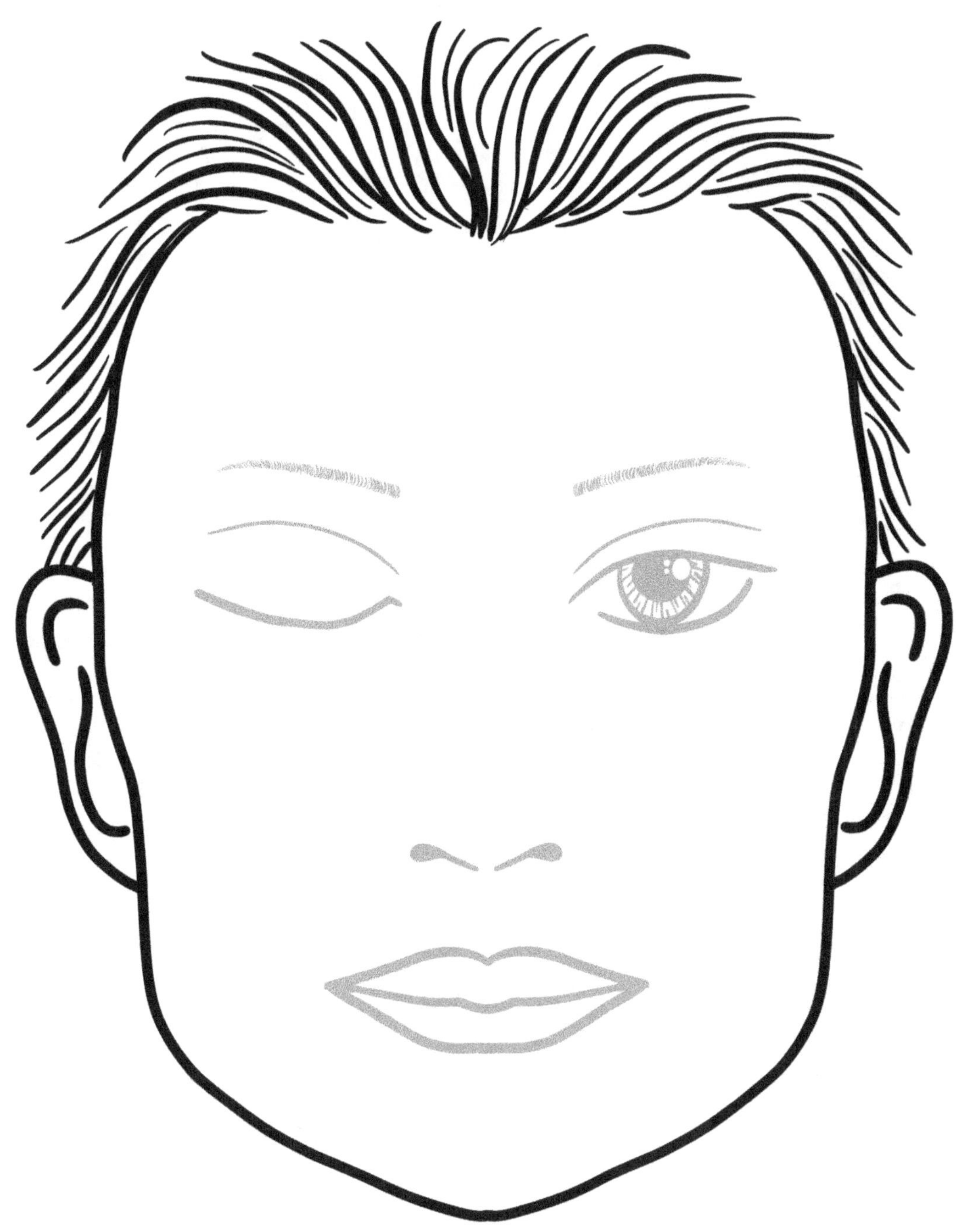

Details

Skin Tone _______________________

Eye Color ______________________

Hair Color _______________________

Lips (color, brand, etc.)

Lip Liner _______________________

Lip Color _______________________

Gloss _______________________

Eyes (color, brand, etc.)

Brows _______________________

Lid Color 1 _______________________

Lid Color 2 _______________________

Lid Color 3 _______________________

Crease _______________________

Eye Liner _______________________

Mascara _______________________

Face (color, brand, etc.)

Concealer _______________________

Foundation _______________________

Contour _______________________

Blush _______________________

Highlights _______________________

Powder _______________________

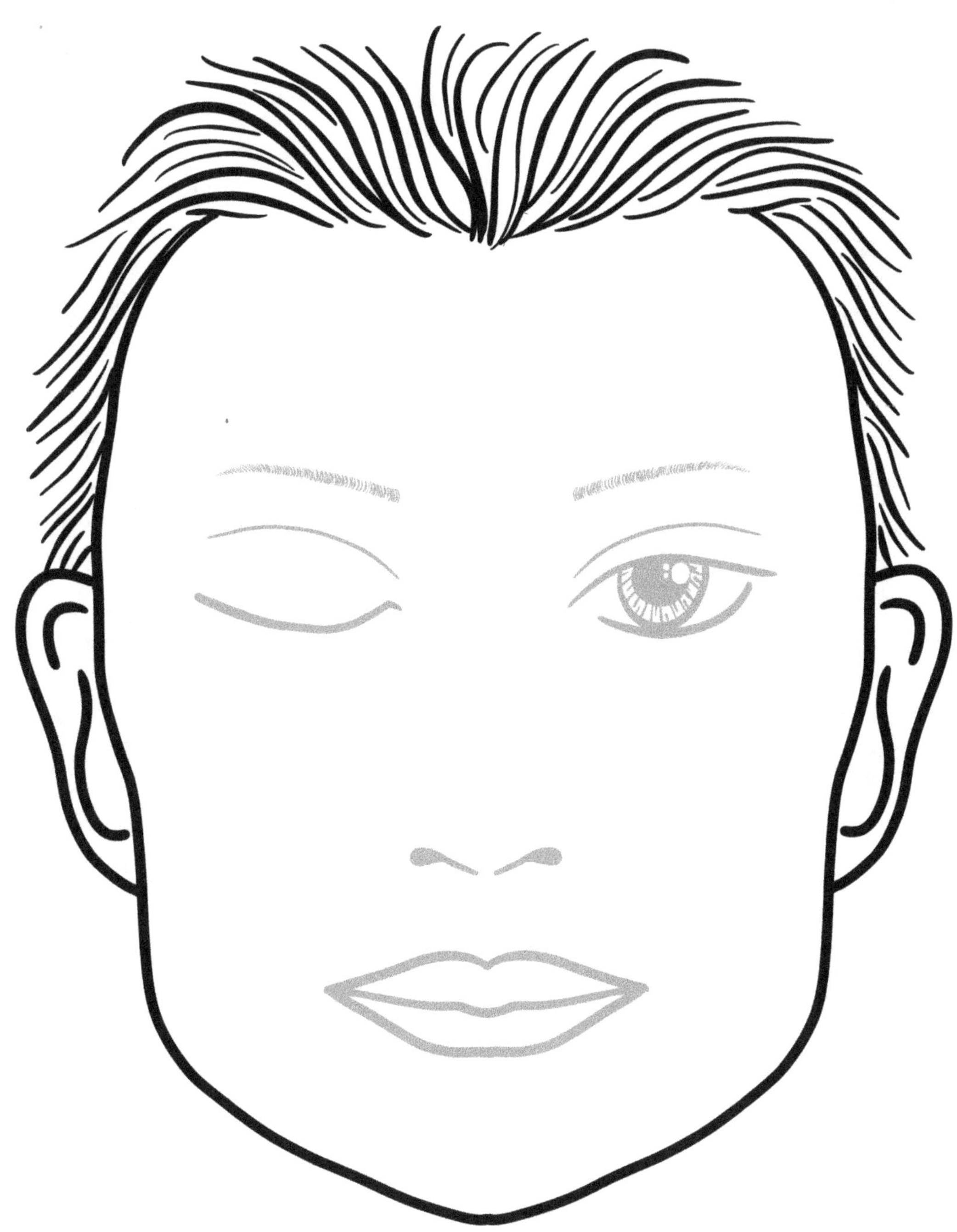

Details

Skin Tone __________________

Eye Color __________________

Hair Color __________________

Lips (color, brand, etc.)

Lip Liner __________________

Lip Color __________________

Gloss __________________

Eyes (color, brand, etc.)

Brows __________________

Lid Color 1 __________________

Lid Color 2 __________________

Lid Color 3 __________________

Crease __________________

Eye Liner __________________

Mascara __________________

Face (color, brand, etc.)

Concealer __________________

Foundation __________________

Contour __________________

Blush __________________

Highlights __________________

Powder __________________

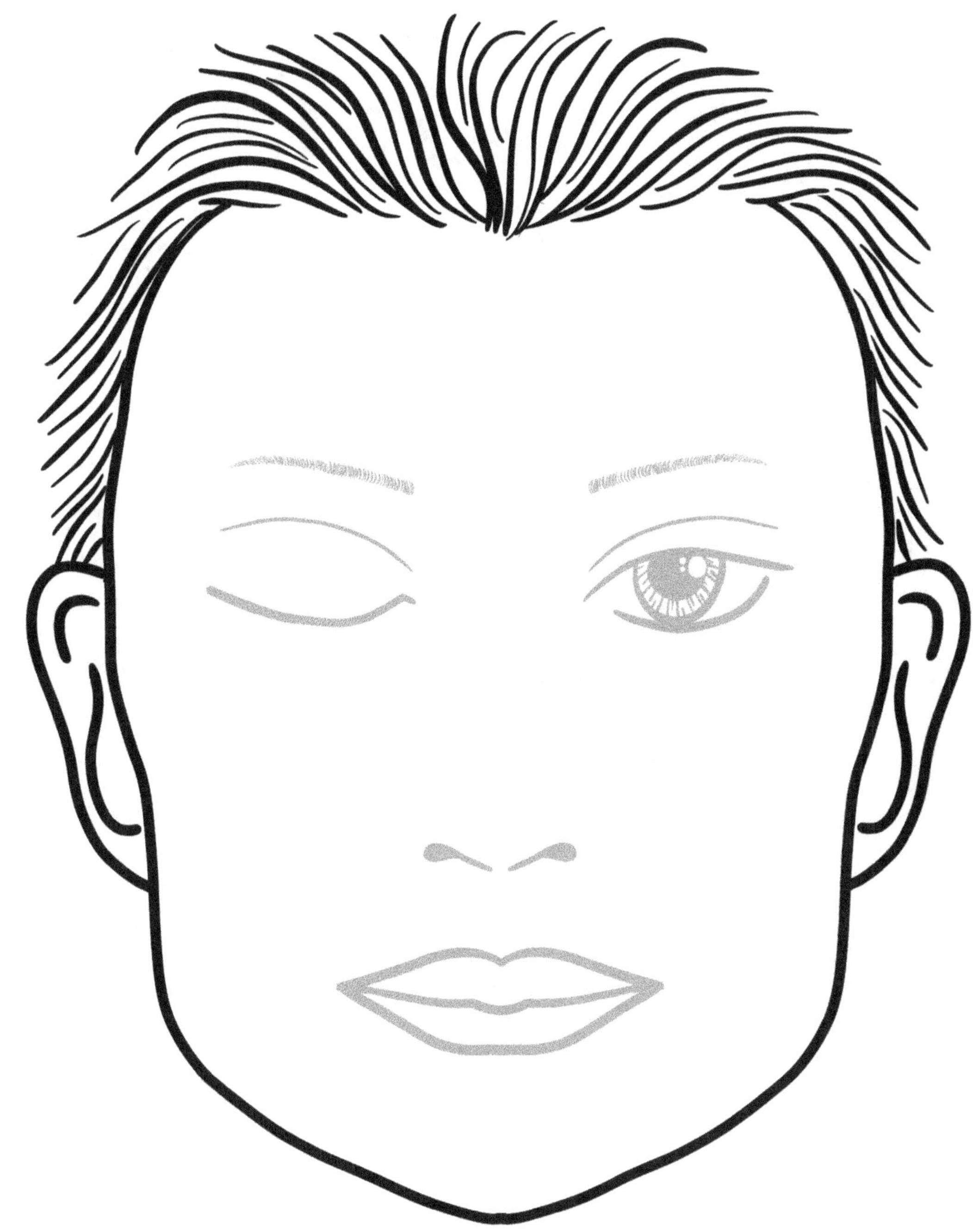

Details

Skin Tone __________________

Eye Color __________________

Hair Color __________________

Lips (color, brand, etc.)

Lip Liner __________________

Lip Color __________________

Gloss __________________

Eyes (color, brand, etc.)

Brows __________________

Lid Color 1 __________________

Lid Color 2 __________________

Lid Color 3 __________________

Crease __________________

Eye Liner __________________

Mascara __________________

Face (color, brand, etc.)

Concealer __________________

Foundation __________________

Contour __________________

Blush __________________

Highlights __________________

Powder __________________

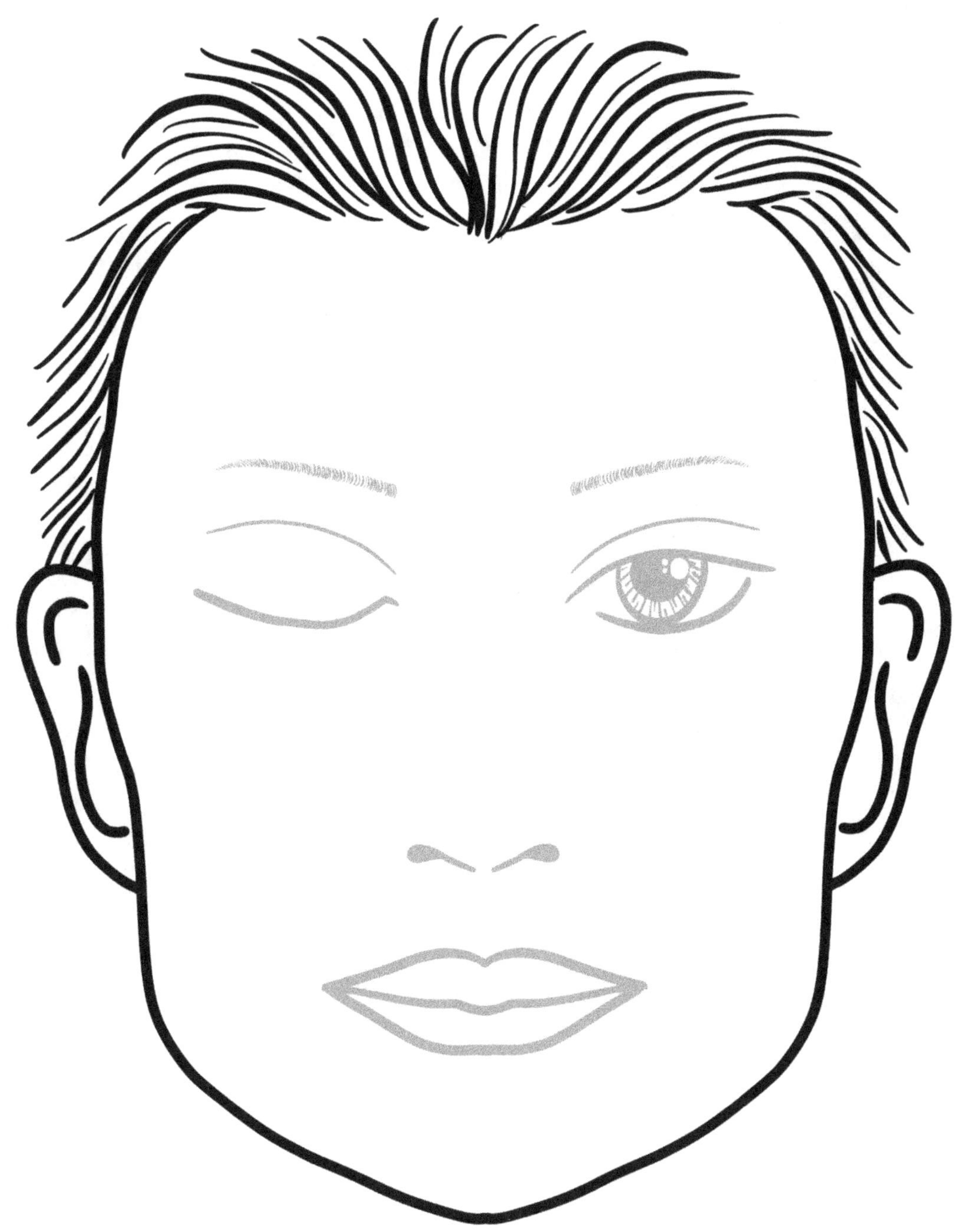

Details

Skin Tone ____________________

Eye Color ____________________

Hair Color ____________________

Lips (color, brand, etc.)

Lip Liner ____________________

Lip Color ____________________

Gloss ____________________

Eyes (color, brand, etc.)

Brows ____________________

Lid Color 1 ____________________

Lid Color 2 ____________________

Lid Color 3 ____________________

Crease ____________________

Eye Liner ____________________

Mascara ____________________

Face (color, brand, etc.)

Concealer ____________________

Foundation ____________________

Contour ____________________

Blush ____________________

Highlights ____________________

Powder ____________________

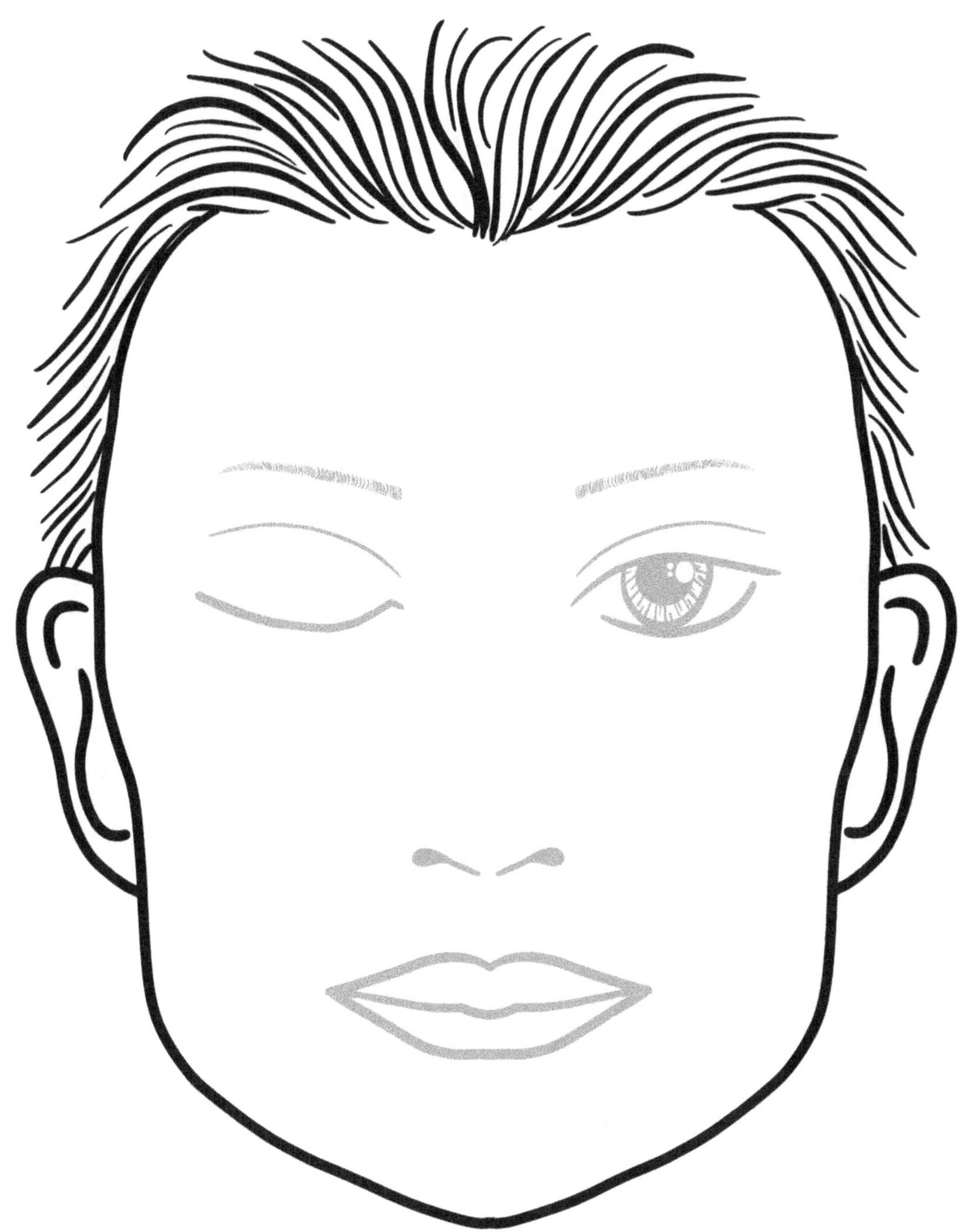

Date

Design/Client Name

| Concealer | Foundation | Contour | Blush | Highlights | Powder | Eye Liner | Mascara |
| Brows | Lid Color 1 | Lid Color 2 | Lid Color 3 | Crease | Lip Liner | Lip Color | Lip Gloss |

Details

Skin Tone _______________________

Eye Color _______________________

Hair Color _______________________

Lips (color, brand, etc.)

Lip Liner _______________________

Lip Color _______________________

Gloss _______________________

Eyes (color, brand, etc.)

Brows _______________________

Lid Color 1 _______________________

Lid Color 2 _______________________

Lid Color 3 _______________________

Crease _______________________

Eye Liner _______________________

Mascara _______________________

Face (color, brand, etc.)

Concealer _______________________

Foundation _______________________

Contour _______________________

Blush _______________________

Highlights _______________________

Powder _______________________

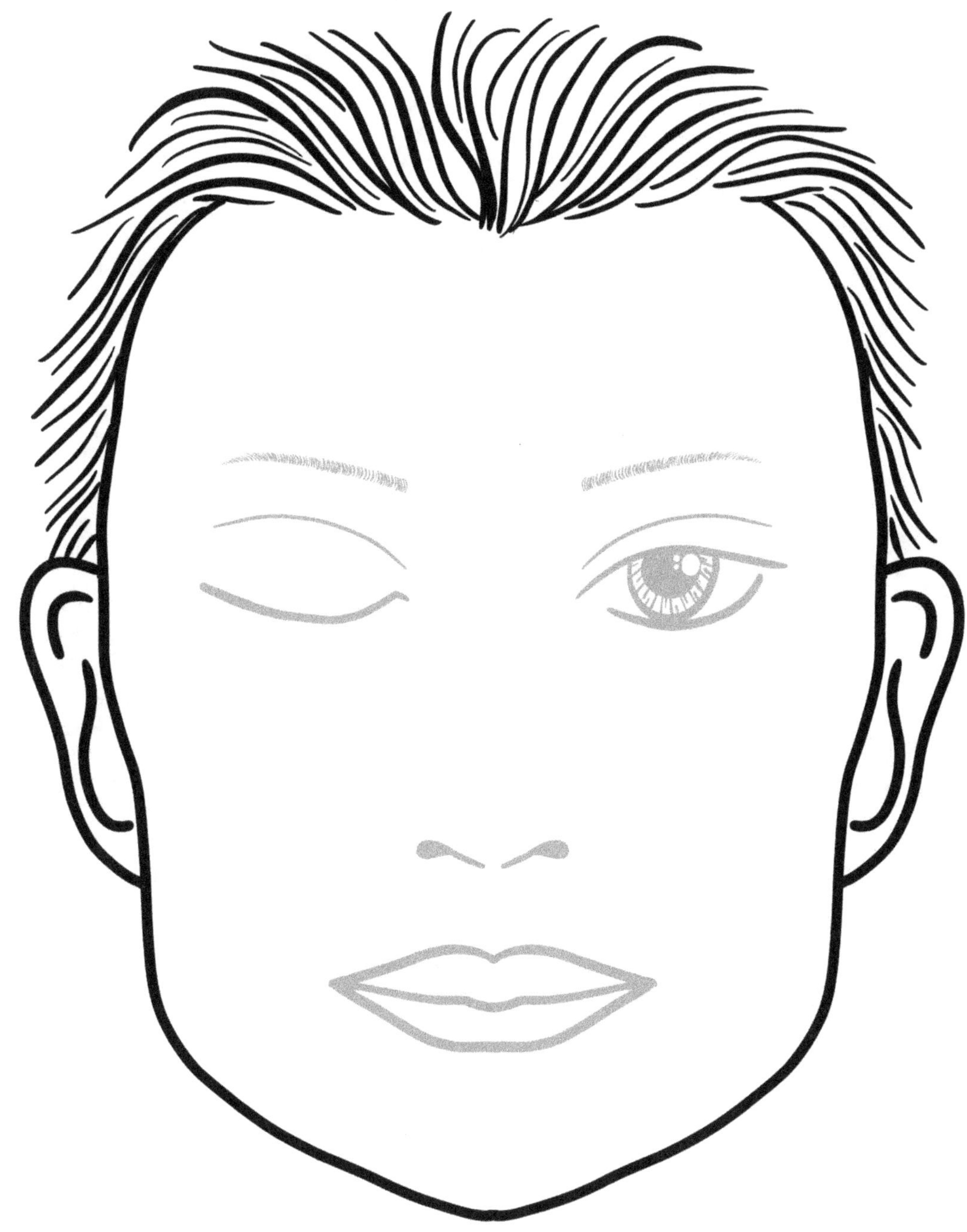

Details

Skin Tone _____________________

Eye Color _____________________

Hair Color _____________________

Lips (color, brand, etc.)

Lip Liner _____________________

Lip Color _____________________

Gloss _____________________

Eyes (color, brand, etc.)

Brows _____________________

Lid Color 1 _____________________

Lid Color 2 _____________________

Lid Color 3 _____________________

Crease _____________________

Eye Liner _____________________

Mascara _____________________

Face (color, brand, etc.)

Concealer _____________________

Foundation _____________________

Contour _____________________

Blush _____________________

Highlights _____________________

Powder _____________________

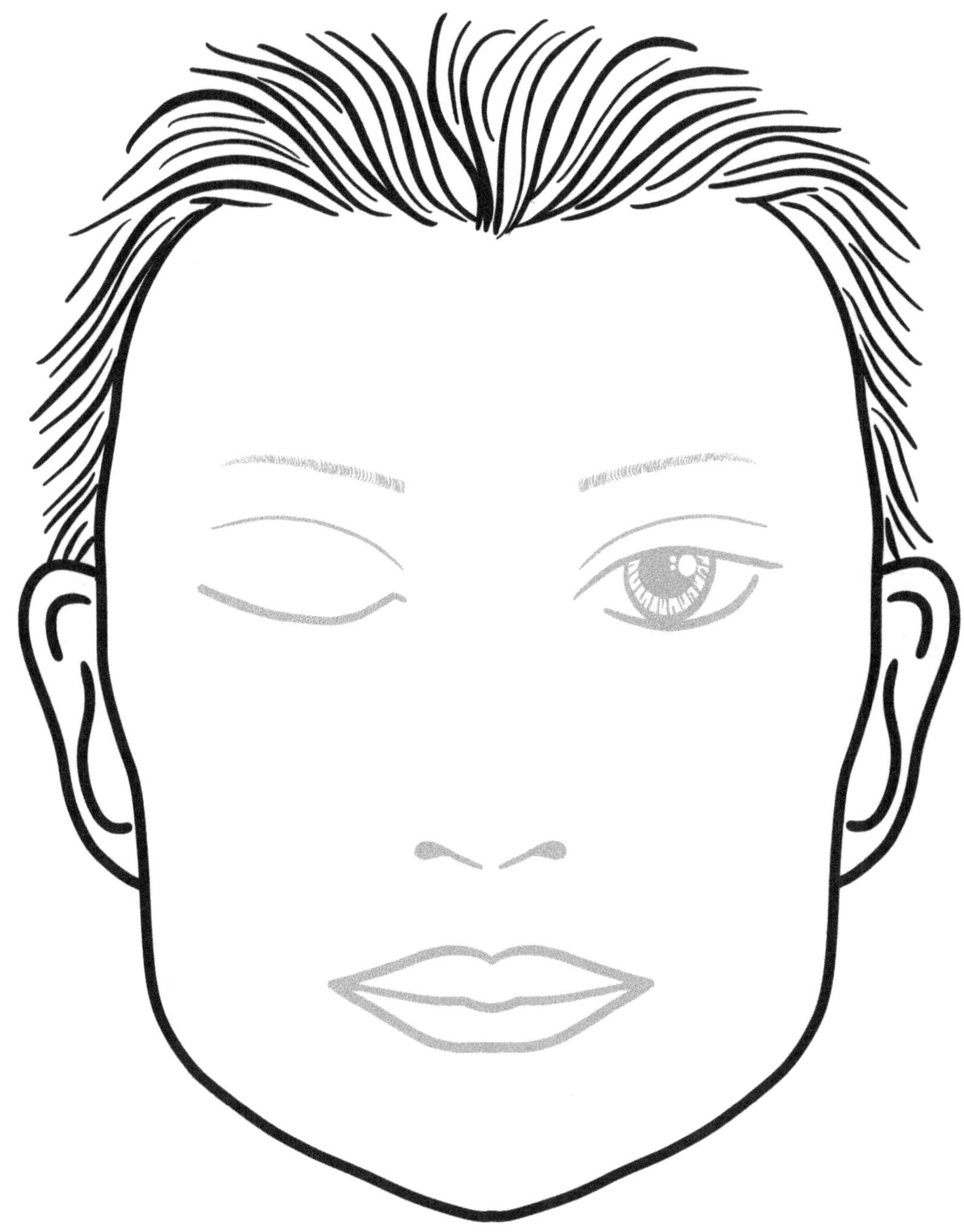

Date

Design/Client Name

| Concealer | Foundation | Contour | Blush | Highlights | Powder | Eye Liner | Mascara |
| Brows | Lid Color 1 | Lid Color 2 | Lid Color 3 | Crease | Lip Liner | Lip Color | Lip Gloss |

Details

Skin Tone _______________________

Eye Color _______________________

Hair Color _______________________

Lips (color, brand, etc.)

Lip Liner _______________________

Lip Color _______________________

Gloss _______________________

Eyes (color, brand, etc.)

Brows _______________________

Lid Color 1 _______________________

Lid Color 2 _______________________

Lid Color 3 _______________________

Crease _______________________

Eye Liner _______________________

Mascara _______________________

Face (color, brand, etc.)

Concealer _______________________

Foundation _______________________

Contour _______________________

Blush _______________________

Highlights _______________________

Powder _______________________

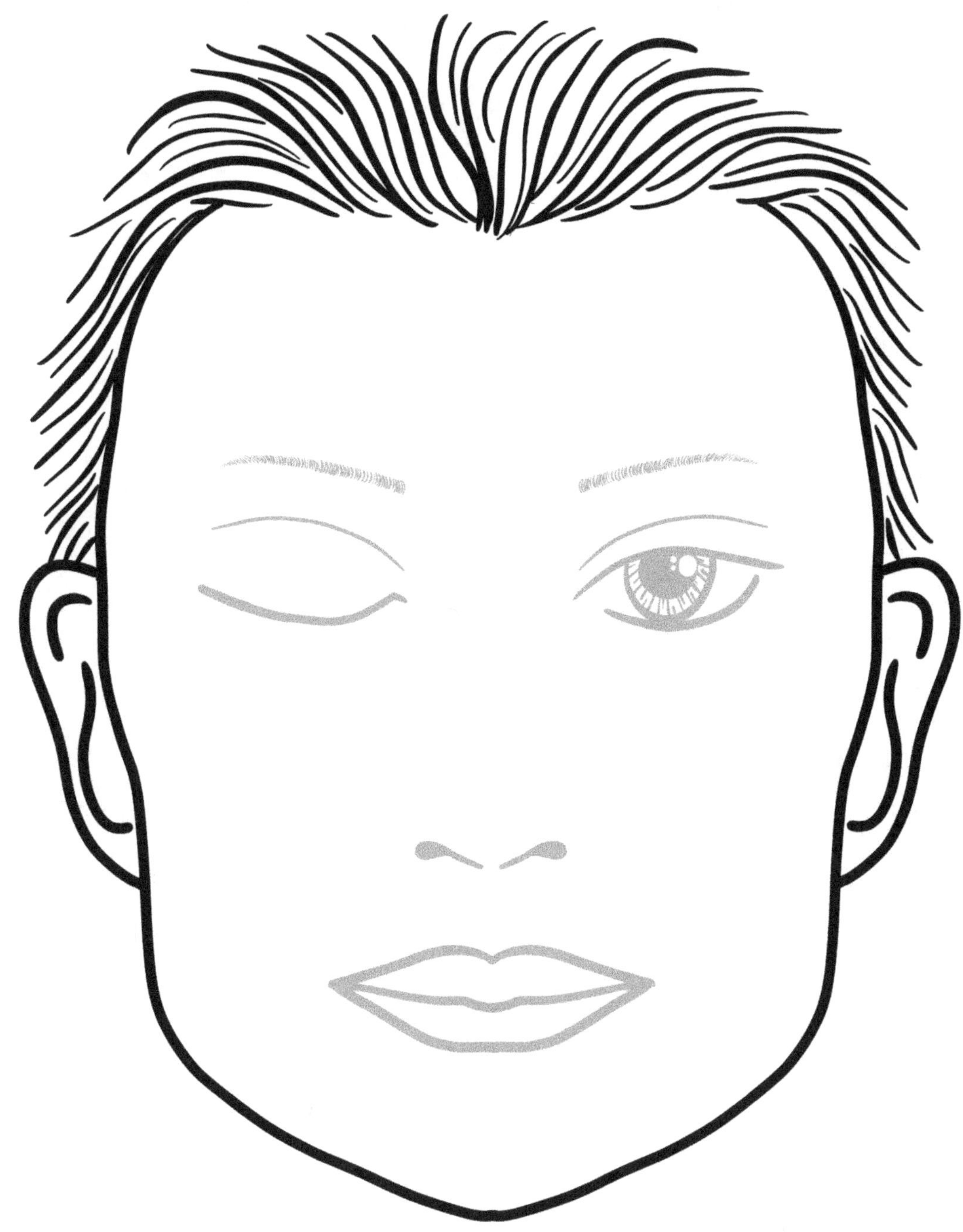

Details

Skin Tone _______________________

Eye Color _______________________

Hair Color _______________________

Lips (color, brand, etc.)

Lip Liner _______________________

Lip Color _______________________

Gloss _______________________

Eyes (color, brand, etc.)

Brows _______________________

Lid Color 1 _______________________

Lid Color 2 _______________________

Lid Color 3 _______________________

Crease _______________________

Eye Liner _______________________

Mascara _______________________

Face (color, brand, etc.)

Concealer _______________________

Foundation _______________________

Contour _______________________

Blush _______________________

Highlights _______________________

Powder _______________________

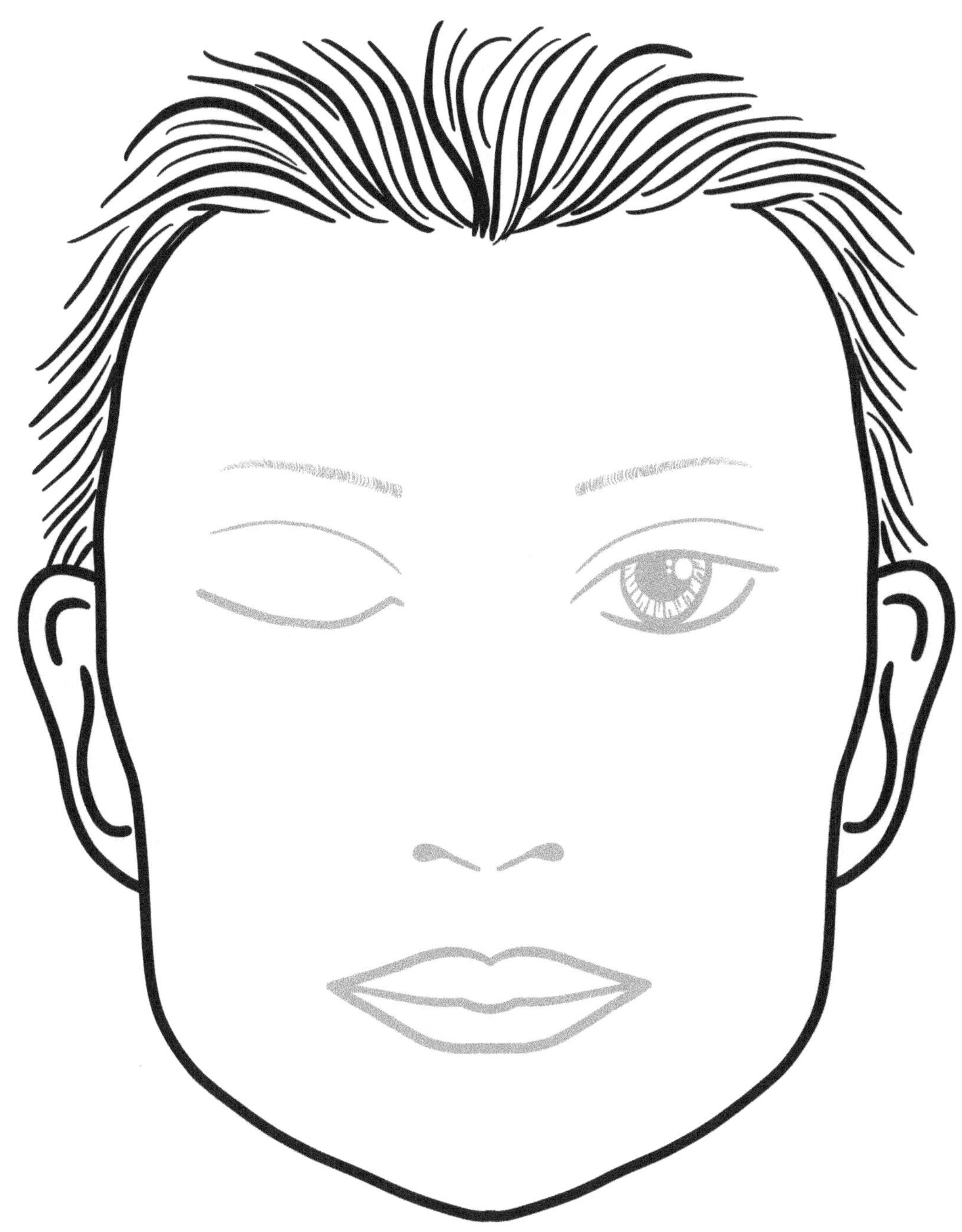

Details

Skin Tone _____________________

Eye Color _____________________

Hair Color _____________________

Lips (color, brand, etc.)

Lip Liner _____________________

Lip Color _____________________

Gloss _____________________

Eyes (color, brand, etc.)

Brows _____________________

Lid Color 1 _____________________

Lid Color 2 _____________________

Lid Color 3 _____________________

Crease _____________________

Eye Liner _____________________

Mascara _____________________

Face (color, brand, etc.)

Concealer _____________________

Foundation _____________________

Contour _____________________

Blush _____________________

Highlights _____________________

Powder _____________________

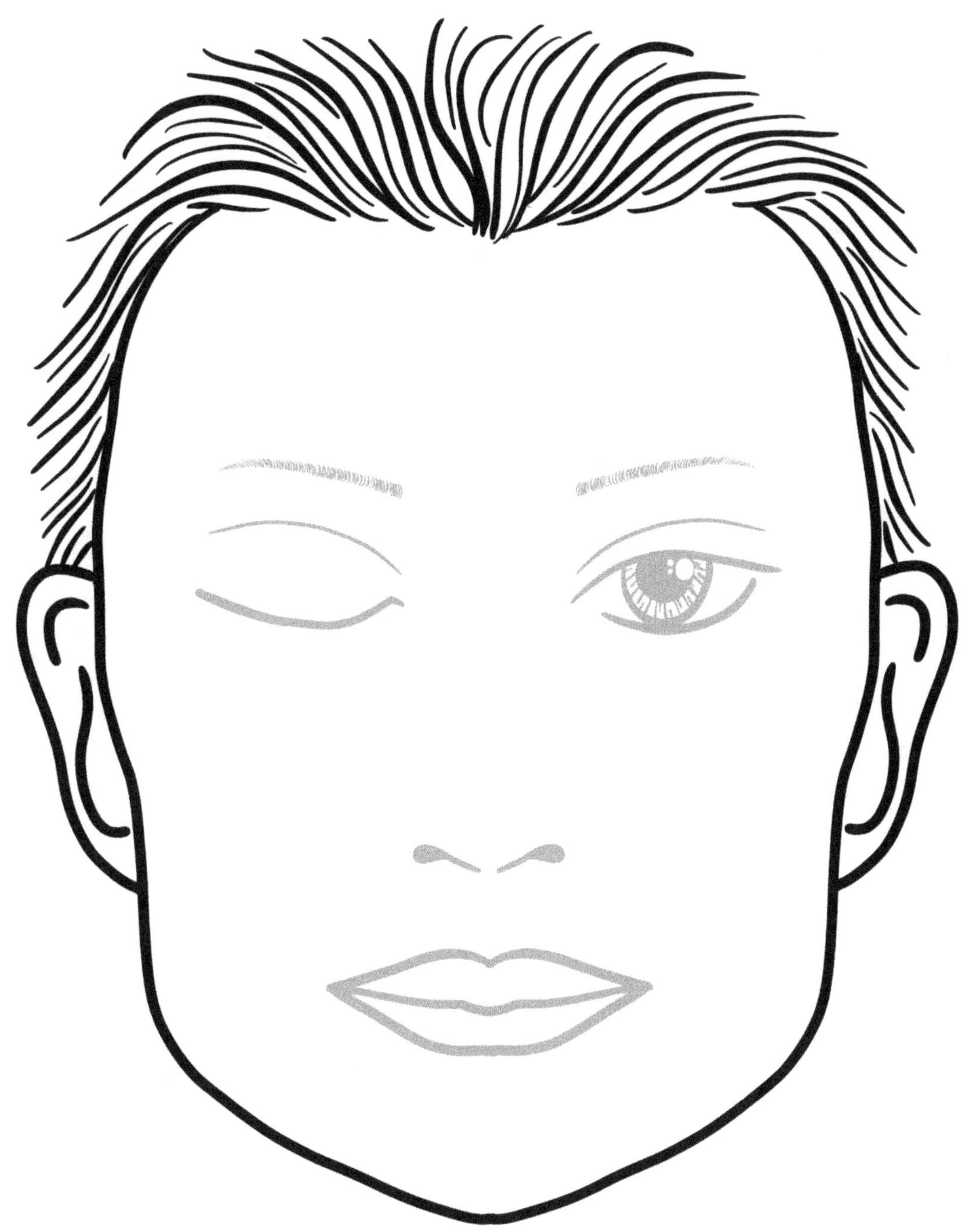

Details

Skin Tone _______________________

Eye Color _______________________

Hair Color _______________________

Lips (color, brand, etc.)

Lip Liner _______________________

Lip Color _______________________

Gloss _______________________

Eyes (color, brand, etc.)

Brows _______________________

Lid Color 1 _______________________

Lid Color 2 _______________________

Lid Color 3 _______________________

Crease _______________________

Eye Liner _______________________

Mascara _______________________

Face (color, brand, etc.)

Concealer _______________________

Foundation _______________________

Contour _______________________

Blush _______________________

Highlights _______________________

Powder _______________________

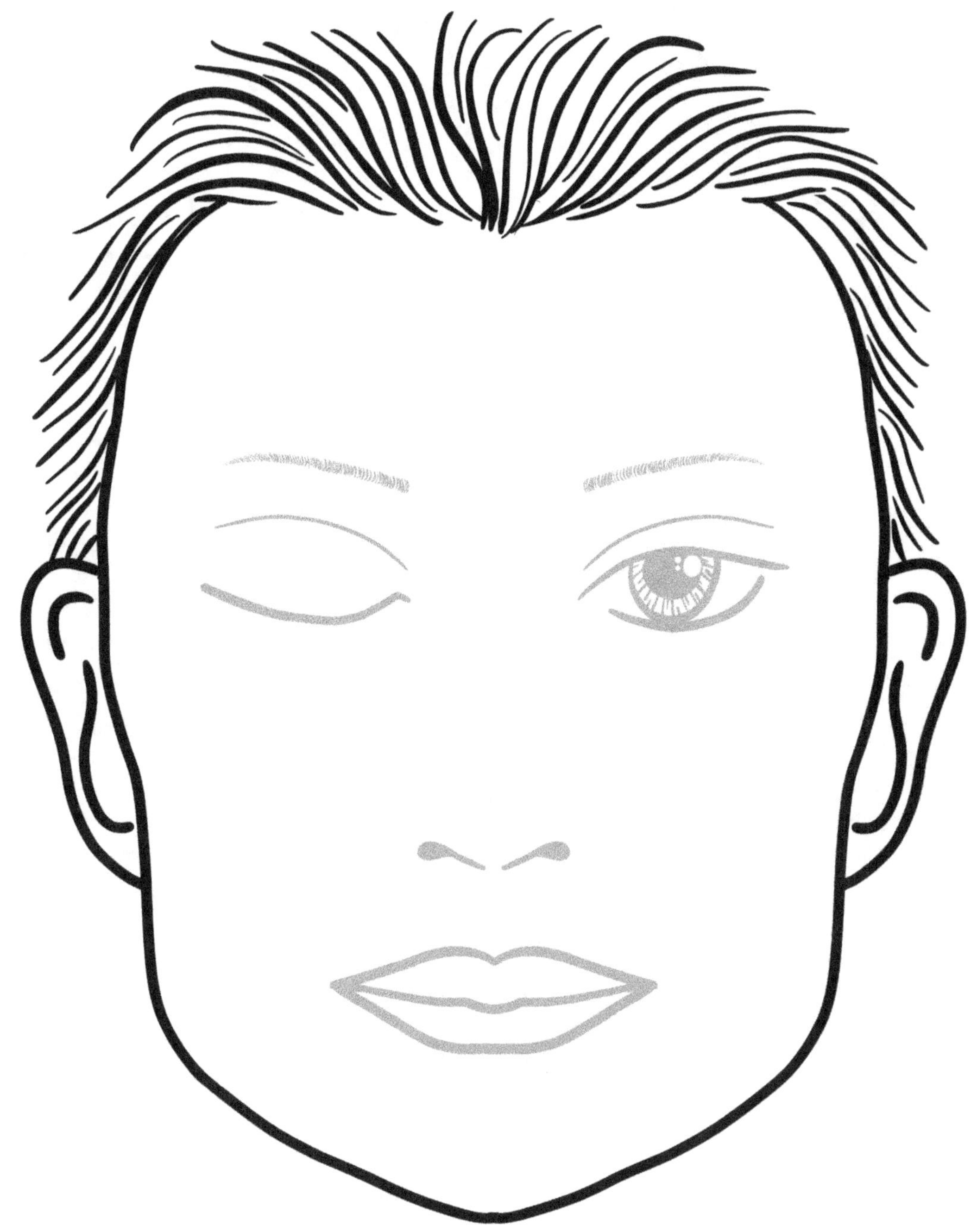

Details

Skin Tone _______________________

Eye Color _______________________

Hair Color _______________________

Lips (color, brand, etc.)

Lip Liner _______________________

Lip Color _______________________

Gloss _______________________

Eyes (color, brand, etc.)

Brows _______________________

Lid Color 1 _______________________

Lid Color 2 _______________________

Lid Color 3 _______________________

Crease _______________________

Eye Liner _______________________

Mascara _______________________

Face (color, brand, etc.)

Concealer _______________________

Foundation _______________________

Contour _______________________

Blush _______________________

Highlights _______________________

Powder _______________________

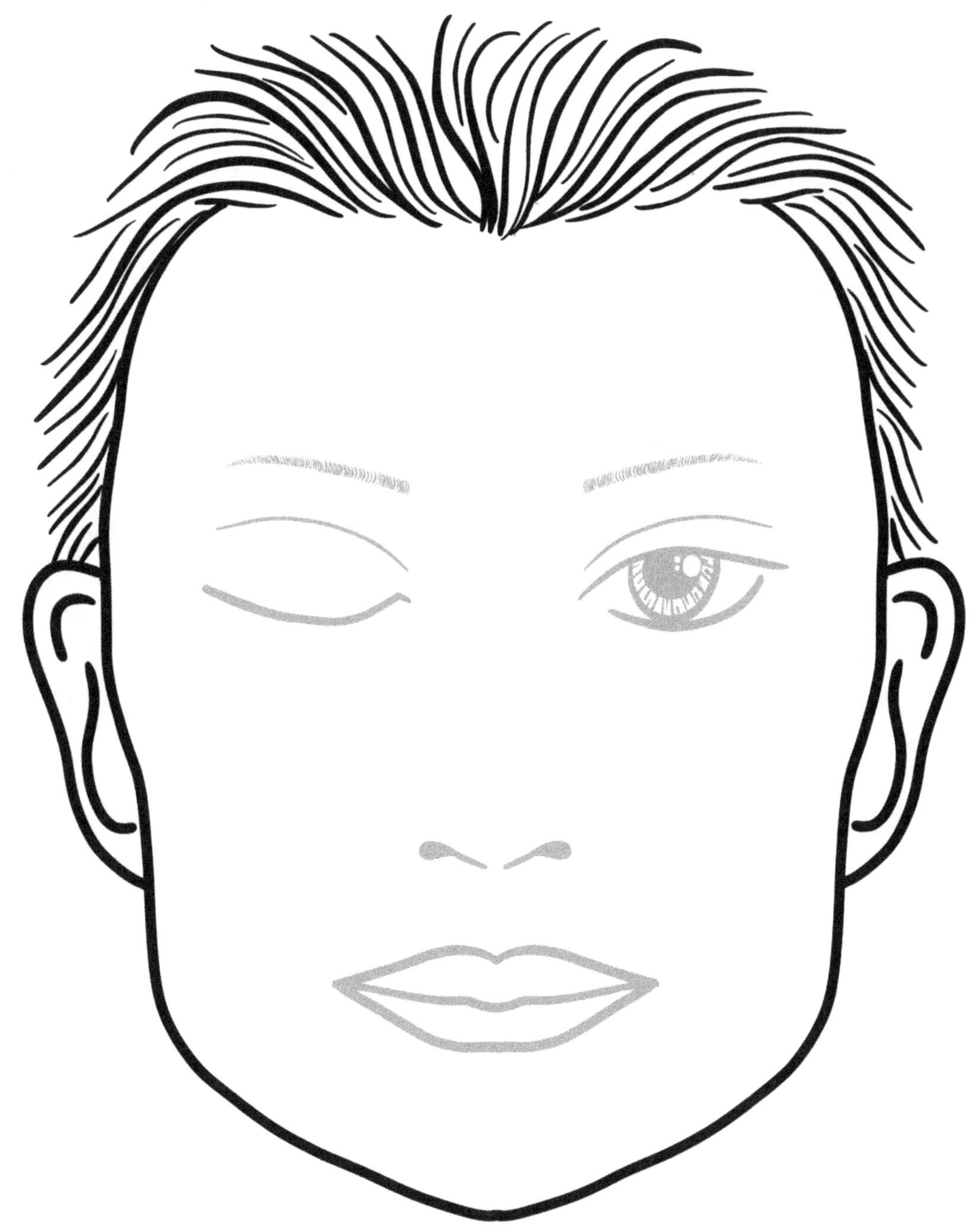

Design/Client Name _______________

Date _______________

| Concealer | Foundation | Contour | Blush | Highlights | Powder | Eye Liner | Mascara |
| Brows | Lid Color 1 | Lid Color 2 | Lid Color 3 | Crease | Lip Liner | Lip Color | Lip Gloss |

Details

Skin Tone _______________

Eye Color _______________

Hair Color _______________

Lips (color, brand, etc.)

Lip Liner _______________

Lip Color _______________

Gloss _______________

Eyes (color, brand, etc.)

Brows _______________

Lid Color 1 _______________

Lid Color 2 _______________

Lid Color 3 _______________

Crease _______________

Eye Liner _______________

Mascara _______________

Face (color, brand, etc.)

Concealer _______________

Foundation _______________

Contour _______________

Blush _______________

Highlights _______________

Powder _______________

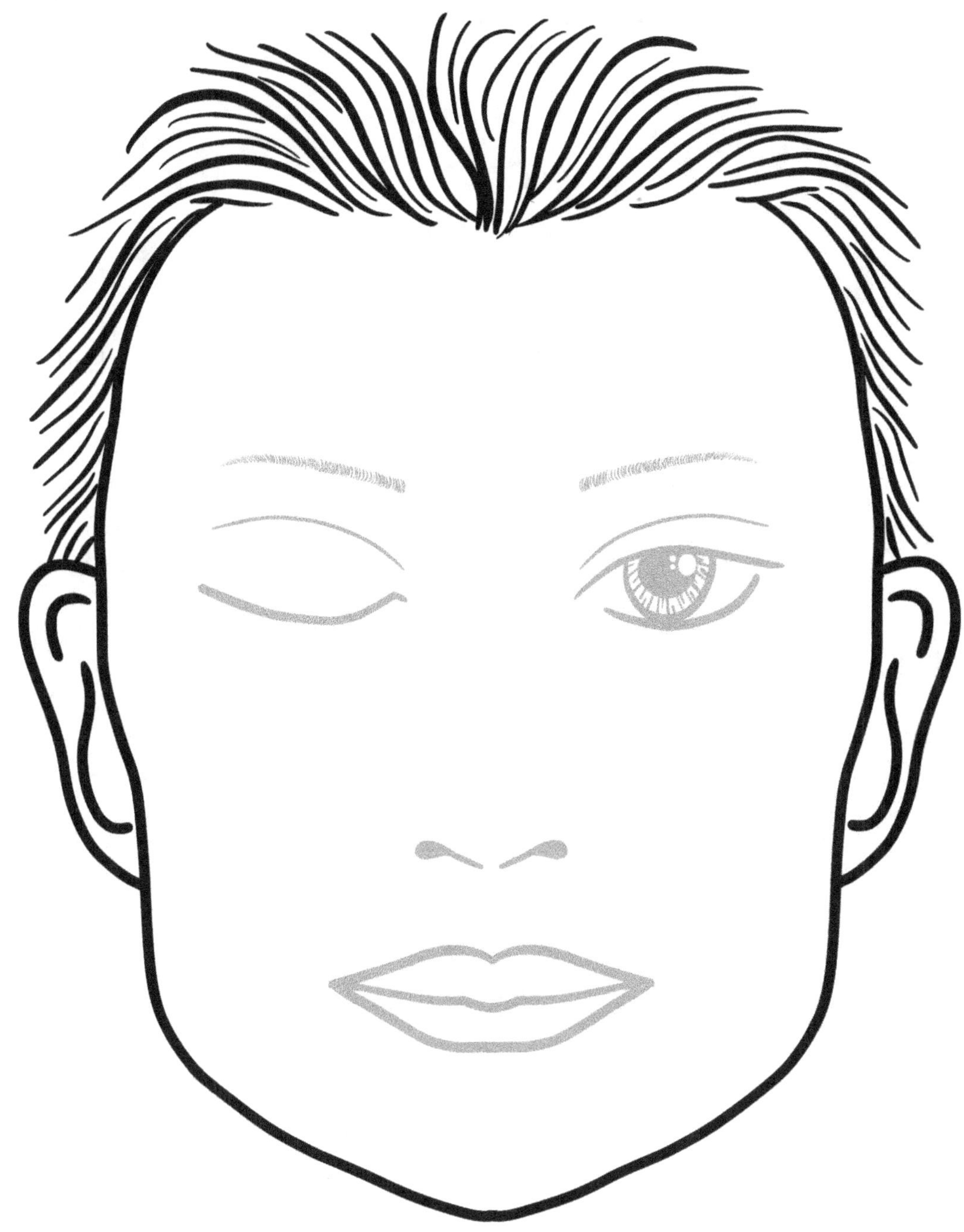

Date

Design/Client Name

Concealer	Foundation	Contour	Blush	Highlights	Powder	Eye Liner	Mascara
Brows	Lid Color 1	Lid Color 2	Lid Color 3	Crease	Lip Liner	Lip Color	Lip Gloss

Details

Skin Tone _______________________

Eye Color _______________________

Hair Color _______________________

Lips (color, brand, etc.)

Lip Liner _______________________

Lip Color _______________________

Gloss _______________________

Eyes (color, brand, etc.)

Brows _______________________

Lid Color 1 _______________________

Lid Color 2 _______________________

Lid Color 3 _______________________

Crease _______________________

Eye Liner _______________________

Mascara _______________________

Face (color, brand, etc.)

Concealer _______________________

Foundation _______________________

Contour _______________________

Blush _______________________

Highlights _______________________

Powder _______________________

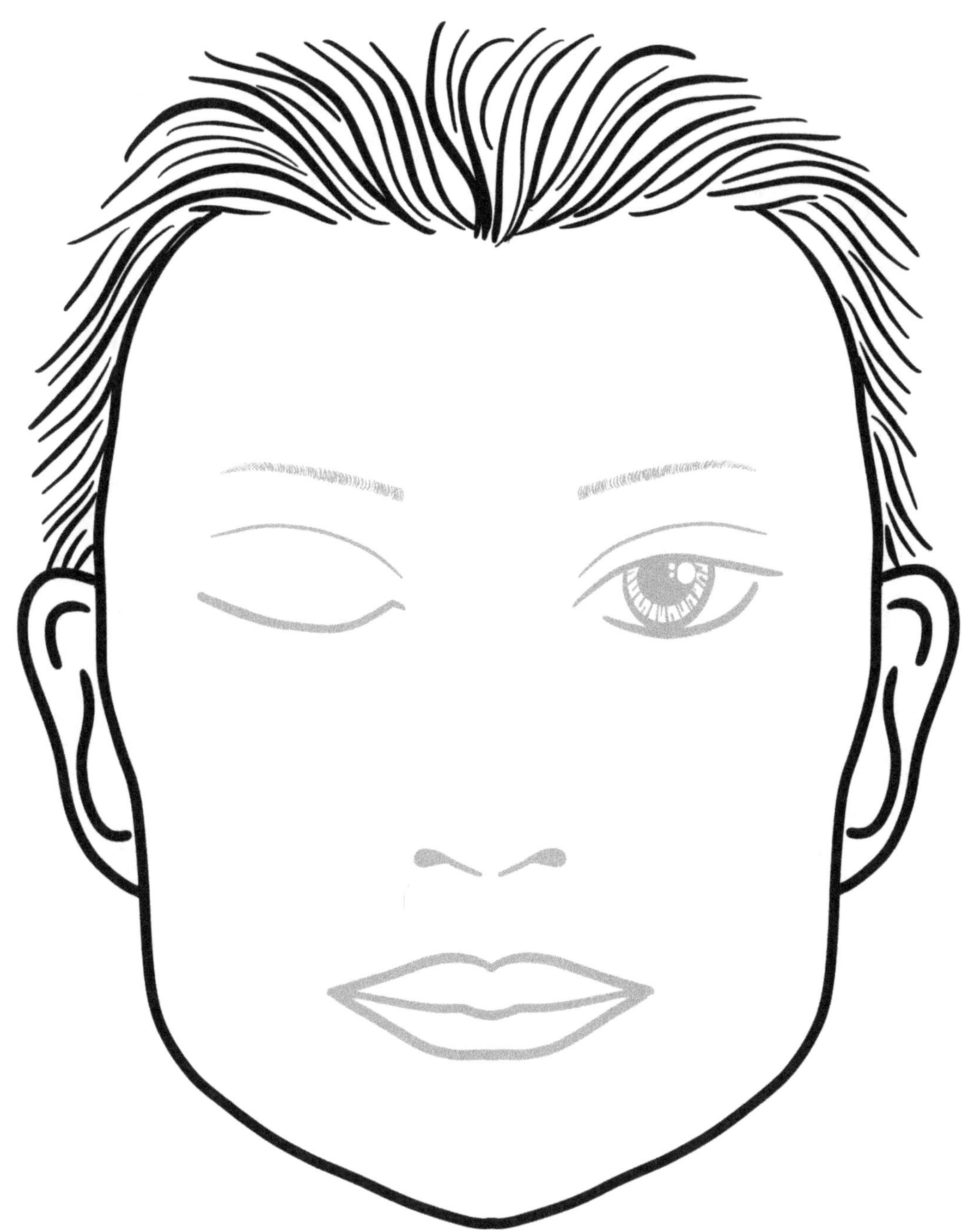

Date ___________

Design/Client Name ___________

Concealer	Foundation	Contour	Blush	Highlights	Powder	Eye Liner	Mascara
Brows	Lid Color 1	Lid Color 2	Lid Color 3	Crease	Lip Liner	Lip Color	Lip Gloss

Details

Skin Tone __________________

Eye Color __________________

Hair Color __________________

Lips (color, brand, etc.)

Lip Liner __________________

Lip Color __________________

Gloss __________________

Eyes (color, brand, etc.)

Brows __________________

Lid Color 1 __________________

Lid Color 2 __________________

Lid Color 3 __________________

Crease __________________

Eye Liner __________________

Mascara __________________

Face (color, brand, etc.)

Concealer __________________

Foundation __________________

Contour __________________

Blush __________________

Highlights __________________

Powder __________________

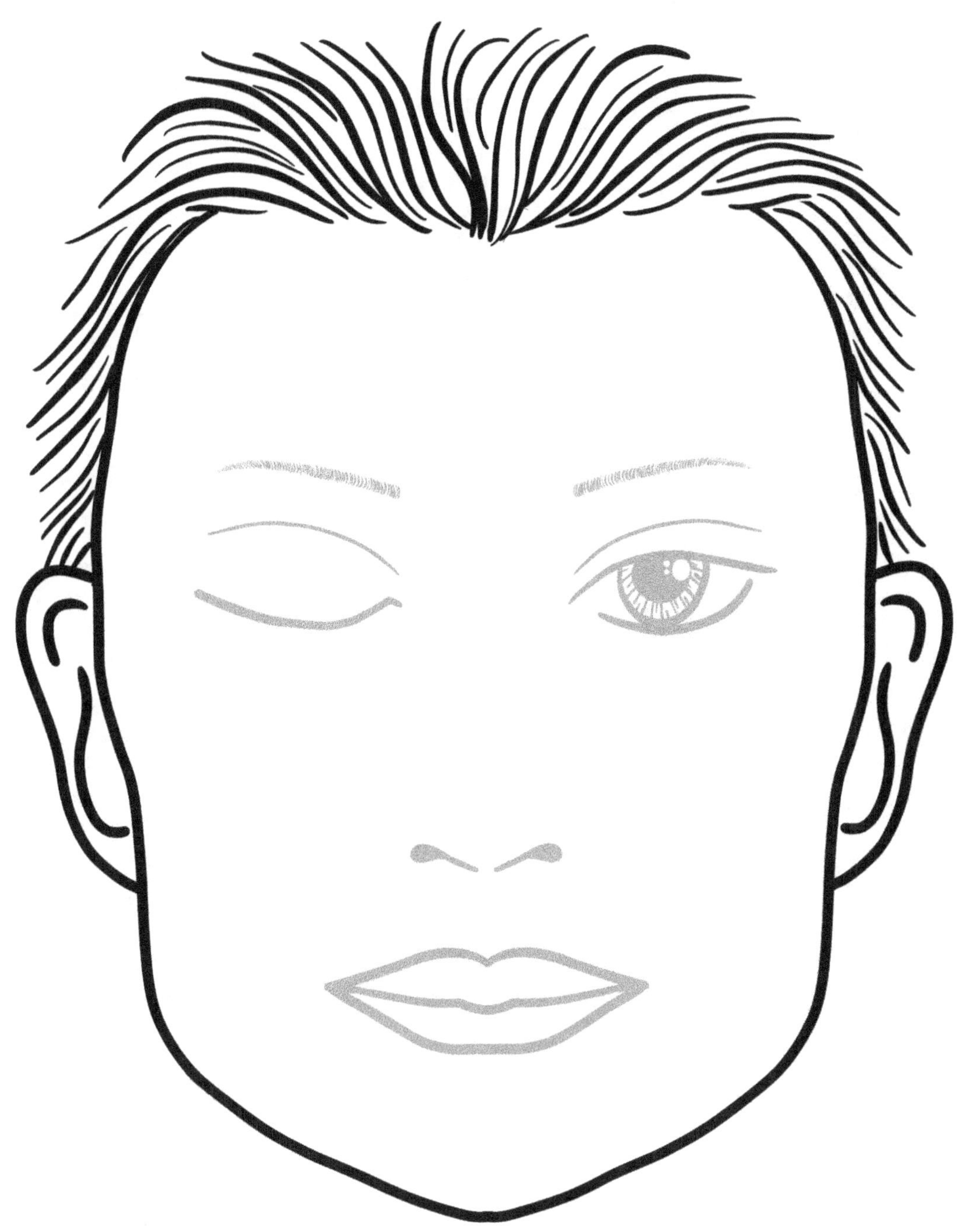

Details

Skin Tone _______________________

Eye Color _______________________

Hair Color _______________________

Lips (color, brand, etc.)

Lip Liner _______________________

Lip Color _______________________

Gloss _______________________

Eyes (color, brand, etc.)

Brows _______________________

Lid Color 1 _______________________

Lid Color 2 _______________________

Lid Color 3 _______________________

Crease _______________________

Eye Liner _______________________

Mascara _______________________

Face (color, brand, etc.)

Concealer _______________________

Foundation _______________________

Contour _______________________

Blush _______________________

Highlights _______________________

Powder _______________________

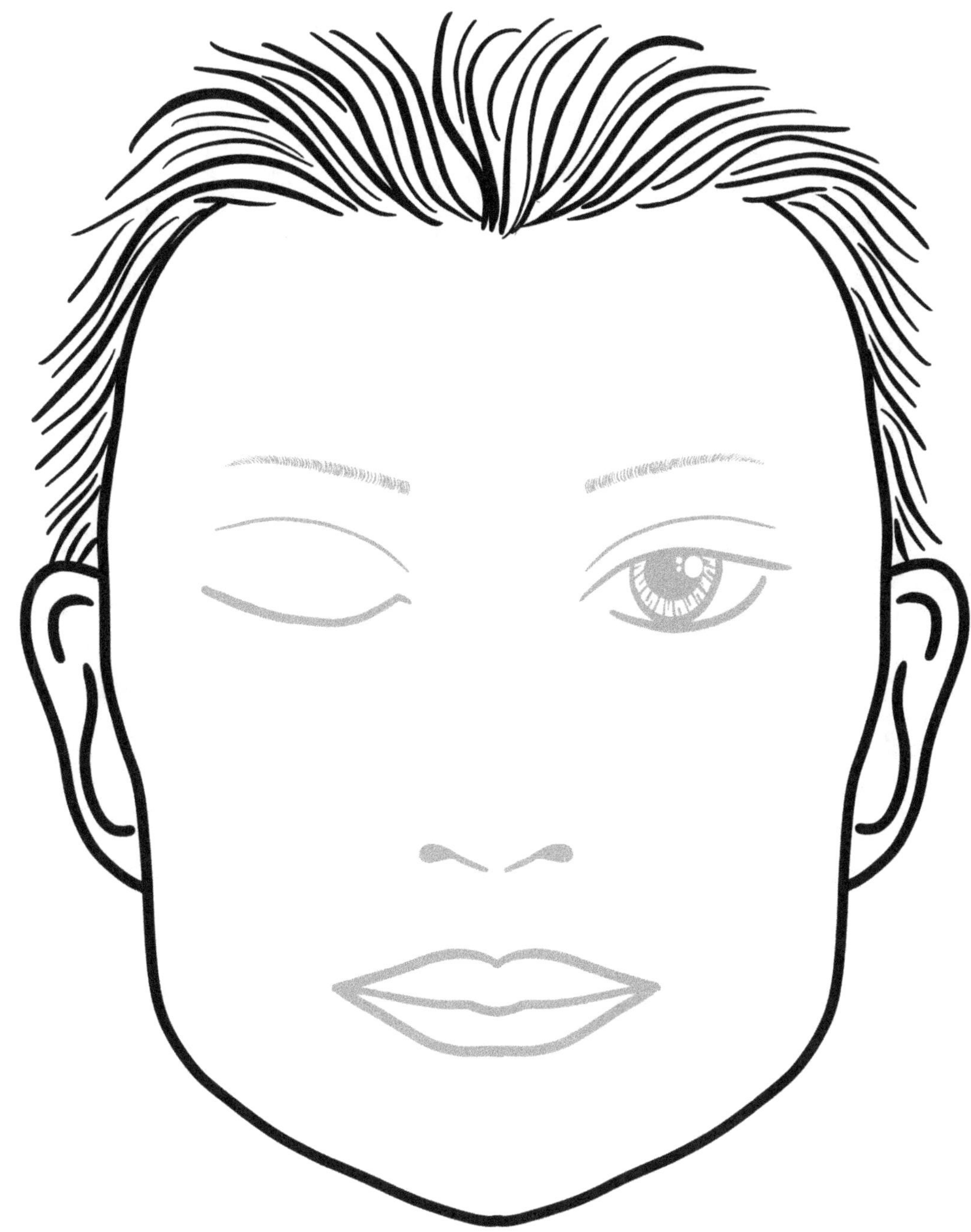

Details

Skin Tone _______________________

Eye Color _______________________

Hair Color _______________________

Lips (color, brand, etc.)

Lip Liner _______________________

Lip Color _______________________

Gloss _______________________

Eyes (color, brand, etc.)

Brows _______________________

Lid Color 1 _______________________

Lid Color 2 _______________________

Lid Color 3 _______________________

Crease _______________________

Eye Liner _______________________

Mascara _______________________

Face (color, brand, etc.)

Concealer _______________________

Foundation _______________________

Contour _______________________

Blush _______________________

Highlights _______________________

Powder _______________________

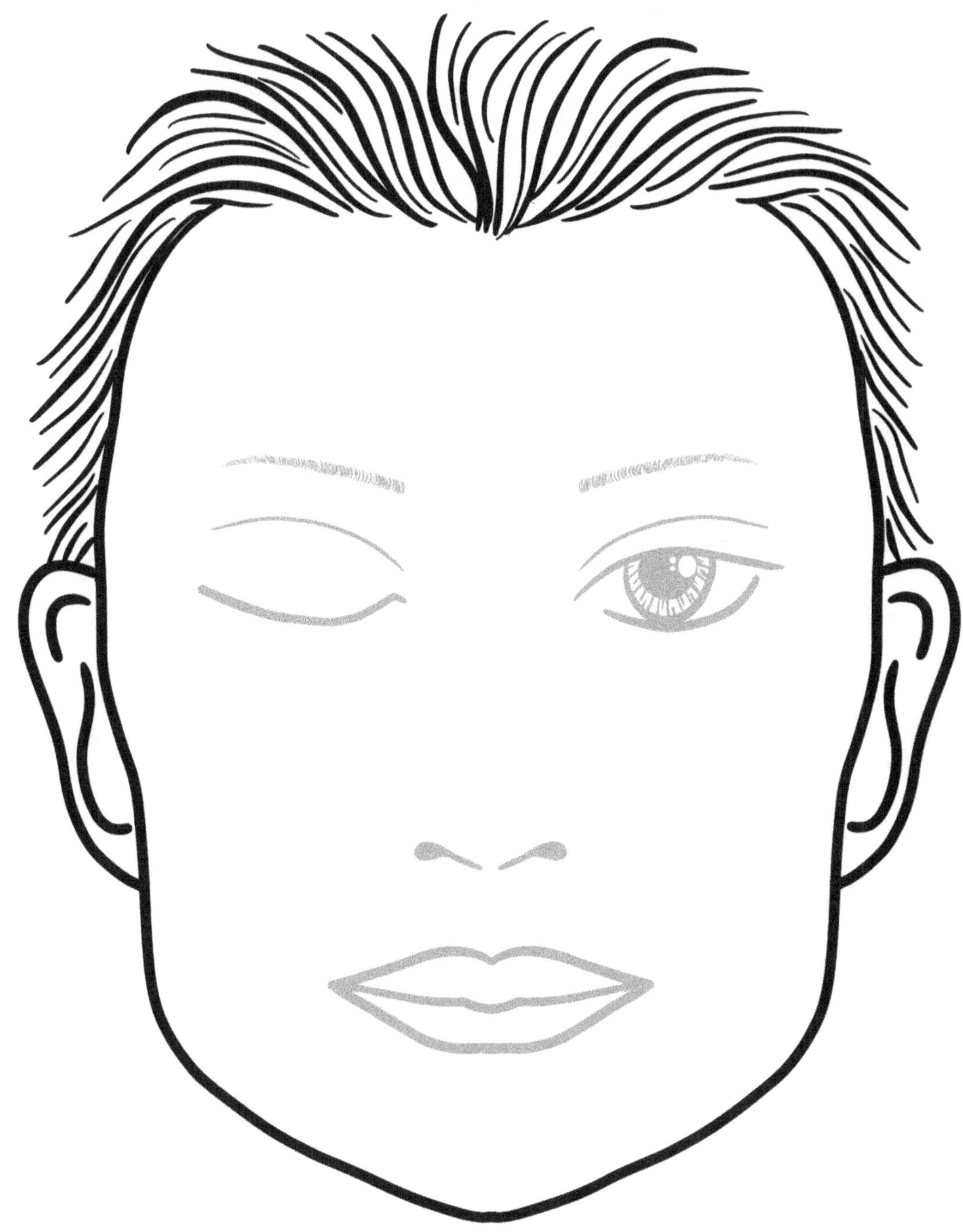

Details

Skin Tone _______________________

Eye Color _______________________

Hair Color _______________________

Lips (color, brand, etc.)

Lip Liner _______________________

Lip Color _______________________

Gloss _______________________

Eyes (color, brand, etc.)

Brows _______________________

Lid Color 1 _______________________

Lid Color 2 _______________________

Lid Color 3 _______________________

Crease _______________________

Eye Liner _______________________

Mascara _______________________

Face (color, brand, etc.)

Concealer _______________________

Foundation _______________________

Contour _______________________

Blush _______________________

Highlights _______________________

Powder _______________________

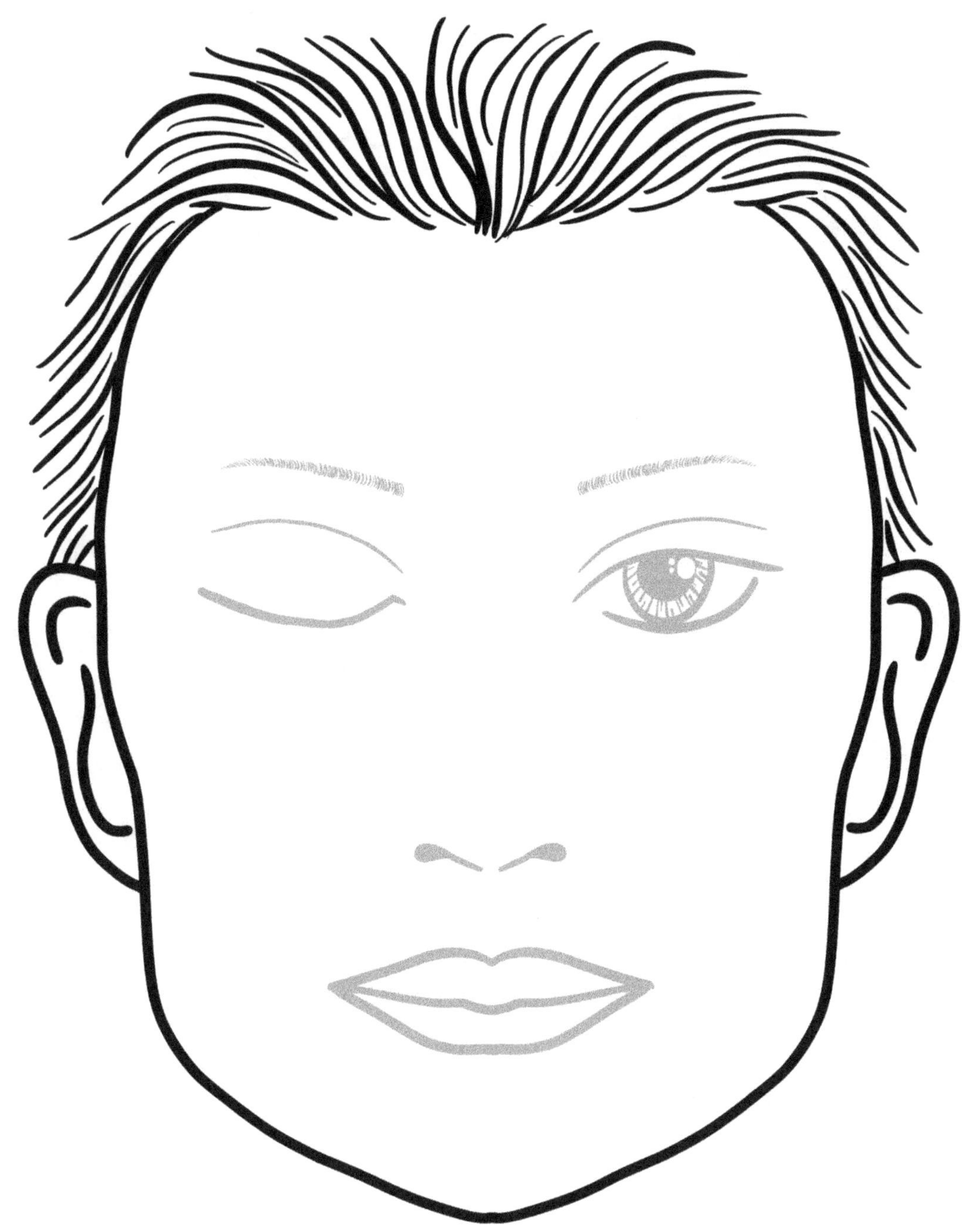

<table>
<tr><td rowspan="2">Date ___________
Design/Client Name ___________</td><td>Mascara</td><td>Eye Liner</td><td>Powder</td><td>Highlights</td><td>Blush</td><td>Contour</td><td>Foundation</td><td>Concealer</td></tr>
<tr><td>Lip Gloss</td><td>Lip Color</td><td>Lip Liner</td><td>Crease</td><td>Lid Color 3</td><td>Lid Color 2</td><td>Lid Color 1</td><td>Brows</td></tr>
</table>

Details

Skin Tone _____________________

Eye Color _____________________

Hair Color _____________________

Lips (color, brand, etc.)

Lip Liner _____________________

Lip Color _____________________

Gloss _____________________

Eyes (color, brand, etc.)

Brows _____________________

Lid Color 1 _____________________

Lid Color 2 _____________________

Lid Color 3 _____________________

Crease _____________________

Eye Liner _____________________

Mascara _____________________

Face (color, brand, etc.)

Concealer _____________________

Foundation _____________________

Contour _____________________

Blush _____________________

Highlights _____________________

Powder _____________________

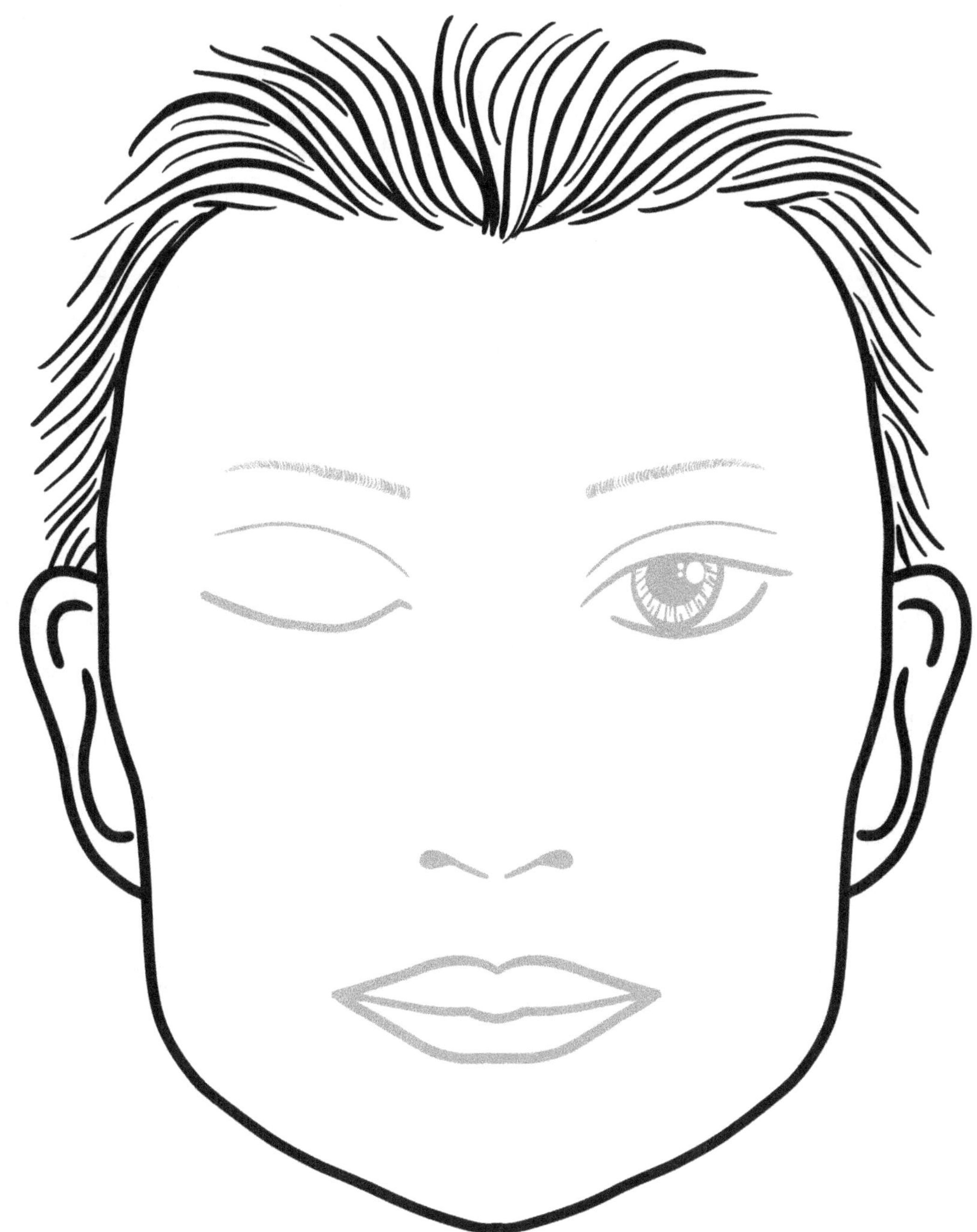

Date

Design/Client Name

Concealer	Foundation	Contour	Blush	Highlights	Powder	Eye Liner	Mascara
Brows	Lid Color 1	Lid Color 2	Lid Color 3	Crease	Lip Liner	Lip Color	Lip Gloss

Details

Skin Tone __________________

Eye Color __________________

Hair Color __________________

Lips (color, brand, etc.)

Lip Liner __________________

Lip Color __________________

Gloss __________________

Eyes (color, brand, etc.)

Brows __________________

Lid Color 1 __________________

Lid Color 2 __________________

Lid Color 3 __________________

Crease __________________

Eye Liner __________________

Mascara __________________

Face (color, brand, etc.)

Concealer __________________

Foundation __________________

Contour __________________

Blush __________________

Highlights __________________

Powder __________________

www.ingramcontent.com/pod-product-compliance
Lightning Source LLC
Chambersburg PA
CBHW081019260726
48662CB00025B/2531